I can't hold on much longer. He's strong as a man. How long will this one last? Deep within a sinking feeling crept through me. *The drug his doctor prescribed doesn't stop these outbursts*. I wondered, *Will we ever know what triggers these tantrums?*

A WHIRLWIND NAMED TIM

SHEILA CRAGG

Vision House
Ventura, CA U.S.A.

The foreign language publishing of all Vision House books in under the direction of GLINT. GLINT provides financial and technical help for the adaptation, translation and publishing of books for millions of people worldwide. For information regarding translation, contact: GLINT, P.O. Box 6688, Ventura, California 93006.

Published 1983 by Vision House
P.O. Box 3875
Ventura, California 93006

Printed in U.S.A.

Library of Congress Cataloging in Publication Data

Cragg, Sheila, 1938-
A whirlwind named Tim.

Reprint. Originally published: Tantrums, toads, and Teddy bears. Scottdale, Pa.: Herald Press, 1979.
1. Hyperactive children—United States—Biography. 2. Epilepsy in children—Patients—United States—Biography. 3. Cragg, Timothy Michael. I. Title.
[RJ506.H9C7 1983] 362.2'092'4 [B] 82-21806
ISBN 0-88449-099-8

To God:
Whose grace is sufficient,
whose plans are
perfect,
whose strength is made
perfect
in weakness.

Contents

Foreword

When the publishers of *A Whirlwind Named Tim* sent me a 225-page, typewritten manuscript asking that I consider writing a foreword to the book, I felt it was necessary to compose yet another "regret" letter. I had received several other manuscripts that week bearing a similar request.

But then I made one critical mistake: I read the first page of Sheila Cragg's book and found myself hooked.

Here is a tender story of a hyperactive child and the family that loved him. All of the raw emotions are evident, from frustration to fear to disappointment to joy to anger, and especially to love.

The author's unusual linguistic gifts are used to pull the reader into her home, making each of us a member of her family. It is a pleasant journey.

I've received hundreds of letters and requests for assistance from the parents of hyperactive children. From today, I'll ask each family to read *A Whirlwind Named Tim*.

Sheila Cragg's book doesn't contain easy solutions and directives, but it certainly verbalizes the agonies of a mother and child who have been there. And curiously, that often helps.

James C. Dobson, Ph.D.
Associate Clinical Professor of Pediatrics
USC School of Medicine

Preface

The words are whispered; their echoes silenced. Hidden. Feared. Misunderstood. It makes no difference whether these words define a child who is crippled, or one who has a mental or emotional disorder, or one with a complex combination of problems. Their plight is the same.

This is the story of our son, Tim, and his thirteen-year struggle to cope with hyperkinesis and nonconvulsive epilepsy. More than that, it is the story of any exceptional child who desires to succeed while his family follows an anguished quest for answers, understanding, and guidance.

Like many parents of an exceptional child, we were plagued with the inner incriminations that maybe we were to blame. We placed the burden of Tim's uncontrollable behavior on our older son, Kevin, and on ourselves. Where had we failed in our attempts to be the parents we should be? This was, at times, our unspoken and outspoken agony.

We found that neither how we reacted nor what we did made any difference in preventing Tim's rages. We somehow sensed that Tim was not the instigator of these odd actions and angry outbursts, but the victim of them.

Tim's overdosed, disorientated drug world was far worse than his behavior. He was taking three drugs, a total of nine pills a day. *Was this the answer?* we agonized.

There was the teacher who said she understood, but didn't. Tim's regression was swift, resulting in educational testing and a request for special education, which was denied. Tim was transferred to a new school and repeated third grade.

A change in doctors, misdiagnosis, and Tim's bizarre reaction to the wrong drug followed. We sought counseling for ourselves and therapy for Tim. Failure haunted, captured, and almost destroyed Tim. Four frustrating years of countless attempts to convince school administrators of Tim's need passed. He was finally placed in special education classes in sixth grade.

There were moments when our faith in God was mustard-seed size, and doubt was close to devouring that. *Why, God, why?* we questioned. Despite His seeming silence and our despair, He steadfastly sustained us. Even during our darkest hours, humor peeked through and lightened our days.

But we are not alone in these circumstances. Parents of exceptional children share much in common. Even though each child's problem is uniquely his own, the family must grapple with certain universal questions almost daily. How do we help our child secure success in a "normal" world? How can we maintain a sense of stability and wholeness? How are our other children affected? What about the stress on our marriage? Then there is the strain of medical bills on an already limited budget, and the need to find adequate education.

Hopefully, we've found some answers to share with other parents, family, friends, teachers, doctors, and professional people. Beyond that, we have a deeper hope to offer. Our faith in Christ, who is our Counselor and strength, is a woven thread throughout the tapestry of our life.

Now, as Tim treads through adolescence into adulthood, it is our hope that his "whirlwind" experiences will be stored in life's hope chest of the past. It is our desire that as Tim grows, matures, and makes life-changing adult decisions he will have the right to identify or not identify with, to share or not to share, this story of his childhood.

For this reason, with the exception of Ron and me, we have chosen in this book to change both our sons' names and the names of most of our family, friends, and other people involved in our lives. Other than Dr. Messenger and Dr. Walters, we have concealed the identities of all professional people such as doctors, psychologists, and teachers.

I would like to express my deepest gratitude to my two closest friends, Leona Ross and Karen Ann Wojahn, who prayed with and for me during the writing of this book. The hours they set aside to read my many rewrites, their Christlike criticism, devotion, and encouragement cannot be measured. I sincerely thank my editor, Paul M. Schrock, for his guidance and commitment to our story. Special thanks also to Dave Malme, publisher, and Jan Rodger, a tender, caring friend and Vision House editor, who saw this paperback edition into print.

Our special appreciation to the Tesdalls, who have been brother, sister, family; who loved Tim as their own and have been there when we needed them.

Most of all I'd like to express love to my husband, Ron, whose steadfast faithfulness, love, and devotion to me and our two sons is the foundation of our family.

Sheila Cragg
Garden Grove, California

1

Tim's Tantrums

Tim sailed up the driveway on his bicycle and screeched to a halt. Our smiling ten-year-old bounced off his bike and charged through the front door.

The air around him bristled with electricity. His eyes danced. His hands churned the air as he mimicked a funny event of the day. He thrust his fistful of crumpled school papers onto the table.

"Look, Mom. I got 100 percent on my spelling list."

The phone rang, interrupting his steady stream of conversation. Impulsively, he snatched the receiver off its hook.

"Guess what? We won our game today," he blurted. "Mom, can I go to David's house?"

"We're leaving for Grandma's when Kevin gets home from school."

"How come?"

"She invited us for dinner."

"Can't I go to David's for a little while?"

"You won't have time."

"I can't come over. I have to go to Grandma's," he scowled. "See you later, David." When Tim slammed the receiver, it jangled sideways on the hook.

"How come we have to go?" he challenged. "What's there to do there? Huh! Nothing. *Nothing !*"

"You can take your basketball."

"I won't go!" he screamed. He doubled his fist and smashed some cookies on the table. He grabbed a book and slung it across the room.

"Tim. Quit this right now!"

He leaped on the couch, rocked back and forth, and punched it with his fists. Perspiration beads dotted his flushed face. A garble of words gushed through his clenched, grinding teeth.

My repeated attempts to reach him were futile. Tim's eyes were in a fixed glare. I didn't exist. He thrashed, flailed, and pounded the couch.

Suddenly Tim stood and in one swift blow he hammered his fist through the fiberboard seat on our wood rocker. I overtook Tim in time to prevent him from shoving another chair over. Tim turned. I was the object of his wrath.

To stop his attack I locked my arms around his, pulled him to our overstuffed green chair, dropped into it, and blocked his kicking legs with mine.

Tim writhed and struggled to free himself. He screamed and seethed senselessly. His body was soaked with perspiration. Incoherent rage totally engulfed him.

Quietly I soothed, "Calm down, Tim. Calm down."

He didn't hear me. I waited silently. Any anger from me would only feed his. Time ticked slowly, five—ten—fifteen minutes. It seemed forever.

I can't hold on much longer. He's strong as a man. How long will this one last? Deep within a sinking feeling crept through me. *The drug his doctor prescribed doesn't stop these outbursts*. I wondered, *Will we ever know what triggers these tantrums? It doesn't make sense. He loves to visit Grandma's. Next time he'll be anxious to go*.

Twenty minutes passed. Finally, Tim melted and slumped

against me. His breathing was labored. It was over. He wept. Gently I lifted his limp body off mine. I went to get a washcloth and handed it to him to sponge the dampness off his face and neck.

"I'm hungry. Can I have a sandwich?" he asked, as if nothing had happened.

I was too drained to answer. Automatically I wandered toward the kitchen. *He's always starved after a rage. He'll be tired and irritable the rest of the day.*

Memories circled through my mind. I was drawn to the beginning, to Tim's birth. I chuckled when I thought about the crazy comedy act that was performed on the afternoon he was born.

Seventeen days overdue, I remember telling the doctor, "I want this baby born today, the twenty-eighth of May. This Friday is Memorial Day and I want to be home for the holiday." It was a statement of pure feminine illogic that only a woman can understand.

"I'd like the day off, too," he reassured me. "You're ready. I'll induce labor, but you'll probably have a long wait. See you at the hospital after dinner."

My mother had driven me to the doctor's office. We decided to visit my mother-in-law, who invited us to stay for lunch. By the time I'd finished eating I was having strong contractions five minutes apart. I called Ron at work, and my mother rushed me to the hospital.

Ron arrived at the hospital and had barely sat down with me when the nurses ushered him out. My contractions were close. I was progressing rapidly. Just as Ron sat down again they shuffled him out and then back in. The nurses were running around frantically. They called the doctor who had to leave an office full of patients.

In two hours and twenty-two minutes our son Timothy Michael Cragg was born.

An hour later when Ron entered my hospital room he smiled jubilantly. Laugh wrinkles surrounded his deep-set blue eyes framed by brown-rimmed glasses. His reddish complexion flushed warmly over his square forehead, wide nose, and cheekbones. His short, stocky build and ruddy features reminded me of the typical Irishman, which was one of many other nationalities that had formed his heritage. He was soft-spoken, an unobtrusive observer of humanity, and was endowed with a seventh sense—a sense of humor.

He bent down, kissed me on the cheek, and gripped my hand as he sat down at my bedside. "Our son is beautiful," he said simply. I laughed as he commented on the three-ring circus delivery.

I was keyed-up and running on pure aftershock elation. "That was so easy I could have another baby tomorrow. It was hardly more than a good case of the cramps."

Ron patted my arm and turned a little gray. "We don't need to rush right out today."

"I'm so anxious to see the baby," I rambled on. "They knocked me out and I never got to see what he looks like. Did you have a chance to talk to the doctor? What did he have to say?"

"The doctor said he was fine. He mentioned that the baby had trouble breathing in the beginning because of a mucous plug in his throat." Ron stood, "Honey, you need some rest. Why don't I leave now. I'll call our family and friends. See you tonight."

When they finally brought Tim to me late that evening, I was thrilled to see that his head was perfectly formed. He had a thin layer of brown hair. His small oval face had a tiny turned-up nose and a bow-shaped mouth. I checked him over closely and was pleased to find that his long thin body was well formed and his delicate pink toes and fingers were normal.

We were without health insurance and short on necessary funds. The doctor released us Thursday, thirty-six hours after Tim's birth and the day before Memorial Day.

When we arrived home from the hospital everything changed. Tim was a fretful baby with colic and diarrhea. I could think of many valid reasons why he didn't adjust. I was tired, had a bladder infection, and my recovery was slow. Kevin, his active two-year-old brother, was at the get-into and self-asserting stage. All the strain, I decided, explained why Tim was inconsolable.

Three months edged into five and we began to realize Tim was not going to outgrow this colic. We tiptoed while he was sleeping because he'd jerk and jump awake at the slightest sound. He raged and cried uncontrollably. Any attempt to soothe him, such as rocking, feeding, and changing diapers was futile.

It was the church nursery attendant who first labeled his angry crying. "He's been having a tantrum. I can't do anything to calm him." Her usual patient ways had been tested beyond endurance. We had no inkling of the significance of these tantrums or the almost twelve-year search that lay ahead before a definite diagnosis, exact causes, and some solutions would be clearly pinpointed.

We consulted our family doctor about Tim's colic. He felt I was nervous, should quit breast-feeding, and put Tim on a bottle. I went home assured that this was the solution, and that I should try to relax.

This change in diet brought an unexpected nightmare. Tim developed diarrhea and vomited his formula. We consulted the doctor again, who diagnosed his problem as the stomach flu. Tim progressed as long as he was on the stomach flu diet. When we put him on a regular diet of food, an unrelenting onslaught of vomiting and diarrhea returned.

Tim had far too many cases of the stomach flu, and when he was fourteen months, we knew a change of doctors was now in order. His arms and legs were spindles, his stomach distended, he had incurable diaper rash, patches of dry spots covered his arms, and he couldn't walk. This physical deterioration concerned us deeply.

Ron and I prayed that God would lead us to a physician who would determine what was wrong. We sought the prayers of our church and the counsel of our family and friends.

We were referred to a pediatrician, and I typed a page-long report to take with me on my first visit. The doctor immediately scheduled a series of diagnostic tests.

For Tim, the strange environment of the laboratory became an awesome world of probing and pain, needles and testing devices, fear and apprehension.

The doctor ruled out cystic fibrosis. We were unable to secure one test so the doctor could only surmise by my report that Tim had a rare digestive disease called celiac. Evidently he was unable to assimilate properly those foods containing wheat, rye, oats, barley, and graham flours.

Gradually Tim began to make positive progress. He gained weight and walked at sixteen months. Tim's hunger, however, never seemed satisfied. We couldn't tell what would upset his stomach and what wouldn't. One time he liked a food and the next he didn't. When I took him outside to play, he'd eat dirt, sand, grass, and gravel by the fistful.

We couldn't make Tim understand that he wasn't supposed to eat the sand in the sandbox. I was forever putting my finger in his mouth trying to clear out the latest debris he'd eaten. One morning I came out to find him with a toadstool in his hand. I cleaned out his mouth, but I couldn't tell if he'd eaten any of the toadstool or not. We had to take him to the hospital so his stomach could be pumped in case he had eaten any of the poisonous mushroom.

From then on I tried to remove any dangerous "edibles" from the yard. We kept reassuring ourselves that his digestive upsets caused his cranky spells and that he would outgrow both when his health improved.

The holidays were close, but Kevin and Tim were too young to understand their significance. For two tiny tots, the wonders of Christmas would be teddy bears and tinseled trees. We gift wrapped Kevin and Tim in red and white candy-striped shirts, red corduroy pants, and fireman suspenders.

The four teddy bears the boys received would become

Tim's treasured friends. Each bear had his own particular personality. One cinnamon brown bear had a music box, and the soft beige bear had chocolate brown trousers with matching dark brown ears and paws. The other two were identical twin turquoise teddys with only their blue and pink neck ribbons to tell them apart.

Kevin spent Christmas Day playing with his grandpa's shoe polishing brush, and no amount of enticement would interest him in his shiny red wagon or other toys.

The hubbub of noise and excitement created by aunts, uncles, cousins, and grandparents was too much for Tim. By the end of the day we tucked a tired and tearful toddler into bed.

2

Batman and Bears— Friends or Foes?

The year Kevin entered kindergarten, Tim was forlorn without a playmate. Kevin sailed through his first year of school like a sailboat gliding across a summer sea.

We went to his school's spring conference. Kevin had made a family album shaped like a house. The cover was our two-story duplex and on the second page was a drawing of Kevin, Tim, and me setting the table. The caption announced: "My mother busted a glass. That is what she is always doing."

The next page showed Ron working on a car, which was accurate because our vintage cars were always breaking down. Pancake, our cat, and an unnamed fish were on the pet page. Kevin's ambition to be a fireman was drawn in blazing shades of red on the last page.

Tim was four years old when Kevin entered first grade. By now he had developed difficulties more serious than his digestive disease. Awakening within us was a disquietude that his continued irritability, angry outbursts, and overactivity were more than dietary in origin.

Tim was a paradox in personality—a boisterous bundle of energy, yet soft and sensitive; temperamental, yet a charming imp. One moment we wanted to hug him and the next minute he'd bug us into utter exasperation.

His twinkling, teasing, blue eyes, winsome smile, and warm personality won our hearts. He had a freckled face and his golden brown hair, when lit by the sun, turned red. Slender and pliable, he'd melt into our arms for a few seconds, hugging us in return.

For Halloween Tim wanted to dress as Batman, to imitate his favorite television hero. I made him a Batman costume and Kevin a Superman outfit. Tim's royal blue cape, long sleeve shirt with insignia, pants, and legging-type boots transformed him.

His eyes danced. A mischievous grin spread across his face. He leaped off dressers, out of trees, and down stairs. His feet flew across the ground in pursuit of the imagined enemy. His lack of fear was frightening. I watched him constantly. He climbed anything and didn't seem to sense that he could harm himself.

Ron and I decided Batman, the indomitable television personality, should be banned from our house. We found that all television for Tim had to be monitored. Since Kevin never became overly excited over imaginary heroes from watching television, Tim's wild reaction bewildered us.

Batman, Superman, cowboys, many cartoons, and any other rock-and sock-'em kids' shows had to be stopped. A few seconds of the sounds of gyrating introduction music, or the running leaping heroes, or the rat-a-tat-tat of gun shells exploding the air, or speeding careening cars caused Tim to run in circles of gleeful frenzy, punching and pounding the air with his fists. He spiraled into such a peak of agitated excitement that it took both Ron and me at least a half hour before we could calm him down.

Even though Tim couldn't watch his favorite show anymore, he loved his Batman shirt and wore it almost daily. He searched until he found it, pulled it off the clothesline, or dragged it out of the dirty clothes hamper so he could put it on.

Even when his shirt became a mass of holes, shredded and stained, he insisted on wearing it.

In January we enrolled Tim in a parent-participation nursery school. Although Tim was approaching five he was placed with the younger group of children because the other class was filled. The first few weeks Tim hid behind me and clung to my skirt. "I don't want to go," he wailed.

His teacher assured me that Tim calmed down as soon as I left. He fit in with the group of three-year-olds, but I wondered if he'd be mature enough for kindergarten.

At the end of the two-and-a-half-hour day, Tim was tired, wound up, and starving. Many times I brought his lunch so he could eat in the car while we drove home. If his morning at school was happy he showed me his paintings or chattered about the morning's activities. If all the children were keyed up and rowdy, or a mother happened to scold Tim, or a project or trip was extra exciting, he'd release his pent-up emotions in the car and at home.

One afternoon I came into his room and found him smashing his teddy bear against the floor. He slung his bear across the room, strode across the floor to retrieve it, then dashed it against the bedpost. He stretched and tore at the bear, then hurled it at the closet doors. I reached down to pick up the bear. Suddenly Tim charged across the room, gripped ahold of me, and grabbed the bear.

Raging, senseless speech spewed from him. Dropping the bear, I turned him around and started to spank him. He struck at me and clawed at everything around us. He jerked forward and threw me off balance. We tumbled to the floor. My pleading "Stop! Tim. Stop!" fell on a deaf blank face. He was oblivious of me.

Trying to contain him, I wrapped my arms and legs around him. His face was fiery red. He swore incoherently and struggled to free himself. He was powerful, almost stronger than I. After an hour he fell limp. Still seething, he cried. The rest of the day Tim was edgy and irritable.

Although Tim had thrown tantrums in the past this was the first one I remembered of such raging intensity. Ron and I didn't know what to do or think. We were baffled.

That night, as usual, Tim lined up his teddy bears, stuffed animals, and pillow on his bed.

"Tim, there's no room for you," his dad teased. "How are you going to sleep? Let's put a couple of bears on the dresser."

"No, no, Dad," he begged, hugging as many as he could reach.

When we prayed with Tim, it was hard to tell who we were praying with, Tim or the nightly lineup of stuffed animals.

3

Rags and Toads

One evening in mid-February, Gordon, a friend of the family, greeted us with a black-and-white curly ball of fur.

"Can we keep him? Please, please," begged Kevin and Tim.

"I don't know if you're old enough to take care of a puppy yet," their dad told them.

"We promise we'll feed and take care of him," Kevin pleaded.

"Are you willing to clean up after the dog?"

"Yes, yes, Dad," they chorused.

"Are you sure? You'll probably play with him a week. Then you won't take care of him anymore."

"Yes, we will, Dad. Honest! He's so cute. Please let us have a puppy."

Finally yielding to their pleas, he sighed and agreed, "All right, you can have the puppy."

Jumping up and down Tim yelled, "Hooray—yaaaa!"

Kevin cradled the puppy in his arms. A Cheshire grin spread across Gordon's face. Mission accomplished, he bid us good-night.

The pup looked like a string floor mop. We appropriately christened him Rags. Although Tim adored the ragamuffin pup, he was highly stimulated by it.

"Here, Rags." Tim dangled a shredded towel in front of the dog.

"Ghhhrr," Rags snapped, and a yank and pull free-for-all was on.

Tim gyrated and scooted around the floor in frenzied circles, with Rags refusing to let go of his grip on the towel.

"Swat, swat." Tim touched the air in swordlike motions.

"Yip!" The pup jumped.

"Not so rough, Tim," Ron warned. "He's just a puppy."

"Pop!" Tim dove to the floor, knocking the puppy pell-mell. Over and over a ball of fur, flying arms and legs tussled.

"Pow, pow, pow," Tim shrieked, clapping his hands and jumping up and down.

"Oooouuww!" the puppy wailed.

"That's enough," Ron intervened. "It's time to let Rags rest."

It took several weeks of close watching and intervention before Tim played calmly with Rags. Rags, fortunately, was spunky and survived unharmed.

Because of Tim's towel wars with the pup, Rags snagged the flapping wash off the line. Tim thought this was hilarious until Rags bit holes in his Batman shirt.

"Mom, Rags pulled the clothes down," Tim yelled. "You bad dog," he shook his finger. "Don't you do that again." But Rags did tear the clothes off again and we had to tie him up on washdays.

Summer's hands clasped us warmly. Kevin, Tim, and their friends dug a large dirt hole in the backyard. They played with their trucks, buckets, and shovels, constructing miniature cities and cardboard forts. Nearby was an old rowboat we'd purchased at the Goodwill as-is lot. The dirt hole and boat were their haven of creativity.

One hot day, the sound of happy voices in the backyard

changed to a babble of yelping and hollering.

"Mom, Mom, come here," Kevin yelled. "Look at Tim. Hurry up!"

I rushed out back expecting to see Tim injured. "What have you done?" I cried.

It was a rather ridiculous question. Obviously, Tim was unharmed. Fully clothed in blue jeans, shirt, socks, and tennis shoes he was submerged up to his neck in an oozing pool of mud. Kevin was soaked. Rags' saturated fur hung in mucky brown ringlets. He charged round and round the mud bath, barking his approval. The onlookers laughed and cheered Tim's antics.

"Out of there!" I ordered. "You'll ruin your clothes."

I squirted Tim and Kevin down with a hose, peeled off their clothes by layers, and brought them in for lunch and rest-time. I squeezed and rinsed their mud-sopped clothes, but no amount of detergent or bleach removed the gray-brown dye.

Despite my efforts to keep Tim and his friends out of the pool of mud, he'd turn on the hose, add water, and sneak in. I finally convinced Tim that if he were going to mire in the mud he'd have to wear a swimsuit, instead of all of his clothes and shoes.

Water forced toads, toads, and more toads out of hiding. Tim tucked them on his lap to pet them or toted them around in his trucks and wagon.

"Can I bring my toads in?" he begged at night. "They can sleep by my bed."

"Toads belong outside."

"How come?"

"It's too warm inside. Toads have to live in cool, wet places," I tried to convince him.

"They'll get away."

"You can keep them safe in a box by the back porch."

After breakfast Tim barged outside to check on his toads. Dead baby toad in hand, he wailed, "See! It's dead. All my toads are gone."

"Look in the gopher holes. You'll find some more," I suggested.

Gleefully, he popped in the back door. "Mom, Mom, I found my biggest one." Tim's slimy toad dripped water on the tile floor.

"Outside with your toads." I pointed to the door.

At bedtime Tim asked again, "Why can't I bring my toads in?"

This time I helped him find a larger box, which he put inside the boat. But by morning, the clever escapists had hopped to freedom.

"My toads got away again," Tim mourned. "You should let me keep them in the house."

"I'm sure you'll find them," I halfheartedly comforted.

Back outside Tim routed his treasured toads from their holes. "Look, Mom," he said, triumphantly thrusting his toad over my sink of sudsy dishes. Mud dribbled down his arms and into the wash water.

"Out, *out!*" I shooed. No matter what, it was a daily in-and-out, toads-and-Tim, muck-and-mess battle.

One toad took residence in a small opening under the ledge of the sidewalk by our front door. Every day Tim watered the ground to keep it damp. The toad faithfully resided under the ledge for a couple months.

Evenings when we came home from church or an outing, a delegation of toads greeted us. Before we entered our duplex Tim always checked on his front-door friend.

Nightly when Ron arrived home from work he teasingly asked, "Well, Tim, how's your toad today?"

One Sunday evening Tim's toad was missing. It was late. We finally dragged Tim off to bed before he could find it. "Maybe the toad went somewhere for a visit. He'll be back tomorrow," Ron tried to assure him.

For several days Tim hunted for his toad. When his dad arrived home, Tim met him with a determined look on his face. "I can't find my toad. It's your fault," he accused Ron. "You didn't let me look for him."

"Tim, I'm afraid your toad decided to move away and find a new home," Ron finally told him. "Why don't you look for another one?"

This didn't console Tim, but he searched for new toads in the backyard. I was grateful toads were scarce and hopeful that toad season was coming to a close.

The last week of August, a church situated on the street behind our duplex was having a daily vacation Bible school. It was not our home church but we were well acquainted with the people who attended. I was sure Kevin and Tim would enjoy the Bible stories, recreation, and crafts. It was another opportunity for Tim to participate in group activities before he went to kindergarten in the fall.

I registered the boys early on Monday morning. I waited with Tim until we found his class and met his teacher. I made sure he was settled and involved before I left.

"I'll enjoy a nice morning of quiet," I reflected. But an hour later Tim bounded in the back door, panting.

"How come you're home?"

"I runned away!"

"How'd you get here?"

His eyes widened. "Mark pushed me over the fence."

"The back fence?"

"Yaaa. I'm thirsty. I want a drink."

I didn't stop to answer but hurried out back to see if Tim's teacher was looking for him. I was shocked when I stopped to survey the fences. My preschooler had scaled a six-foot wall fence, dropped to the ground, and then climbed up and over our six-foot chain-link fence.

"Timmmm," a gasping voice called.

I peeked over our fence. There stood his teacher, peering over the church wall. "Tim—Tim bolted," she puffed, "from the line of children on our way to recreation. I chased him across the field. He was up and over the fence before I could reach him. I can't believe he made it so fast."

"I'll bring Tim back," I said. I thanked her for her efforts and apologized for Tim's behavior.

That night Tim informed us, "I don't like Bible school. I'm not going."

We were concerned that if we let him get away with not going he might decide he didn't like kindergarten and run off. Ron and I agreed he should go back.

The next day I took Tim to Bible school, stayed awhile, then came home. I'd hardly unlocked the front door when Tim crashed through the back.

I rushed to the backyard and there his flustered teacher stood on the other side of our fence gasping for air. His teacher was gracious and understanding. We agreed that I'd bring Tim back if he ran away again. Tim finally stayed the last two days and even wanted to participate in the closing program.

In two weeks school opened. Tim chose his own lunch pail. We went together to pick out new shoes and talked about the things he would be doing at school. He was anxious to go and yet apprehensive.

He was afraid to ride the big yellow bus for fear he'd get lost. Once he realized that I would see him off every morning and his teacher would be there to meet him, he settled into the daily routine. He enjoyed the two and one-half hours of play, painting, picturemaking, and music.

One slight problem erupted, however, and it involved shirts. Well, not just any shirt. Button-down-the-front shirts became Tim's target of objection. He had a fetish for certain clothes and only wanted to wear the ones he liked. The shirts he preferred were soft knit pullovers with no buttons and no zipper.

Button-down shirts were the type that most children were wearing for kindergarten and these were the kind I had bought. I was unaware that Tim would so adamantly oppose these shirts. Kevin liked certain shirts more than others, but he realized that some clothes were worn to school and others for play, and he accepted the difference. Each morning Tim griped about wearing his button-shirts. Reluctantly he trudged off to school.

"He'll get used to them," I kept telling myself.

At lunchtime when he arrived home from school one day, he was wearing a wrinkled pullover play shirt and wadded up in his hand was his plaid button-down.

"Tim, what did you do?"

"I *snucked* my shirt," he giggled sheepishly.

Later, the teacher told me the rest of the story. During recess she looked out to see Tim pushing his hand down inside his pants and shaking his leg vigorously. In seconds, a shirt fell from the bottom of his pant leg onto the ground. Tim took off the shirt he had on, picked up the pullover, and put it on.

For several months we had looked for a home to purchase. It was the end of October when Mr. Martin, a real estate agent, called to tell us he had found a home he thought we'd like. *For sale* signs hadn't been put up yet, and it was $3,000 under everything we had seen before. It was a small two-bedroom house located in an older, treelined, country-style neighborhood.

That evening the widow who owned the house took us on a tour. The enormous yard was like a dense forest with twenty-one trees, varied flowers, and shrubs growing everywhere. The four of us peered, poked, and pushed our way through the yard. The boys were ecstatic as they chattered on our way back to the duplex. We all knew that this was the home for us.

About this time, Rags began acting peculiar. He developed a runny nose and his eyes were glassy and cloudy. Normally he slept outside, so we brought him inside and gave him aspirin crushed in warm milk to help him recover from what we thought was a cold. Rags was unable to eat and his body trembled. We continued our home remedies for a couple more days, which was a mistake.

Tim asked repeatedly, "Is my dog going to be all right?"

That night Rags grew steadily worse. The next morning we located a veterinarian who would see him that afternoon. As we were leaving, Tim pleaded over and over, "Will my dog be okay? I love him so much. He's my friend. He'll be all right, won't he?"

When we arrived at the vet's office he told us that Rags had distemper and a 105-degree temperature. We had waited too long to bring him in. The doctor recommended that Rags be put to sleep.

Tears streamed down my face as I blubbered to the vet how attached we were to the dog and how much the boys loved him. Ron gently took me by the arm and led me to our car.

The cold sleet and misty rain that day joined me as I wept and wondered how we'd explain the loss of our ragamuffin dog to our boys. We both sat in silence knowing deep inside that neither of us had the answers. The windshield wipers rhythmically swished water off the car windows, marking time and bringing that dread moment closer.

When we entered the house Tim looked up at my tear-stained face. "Mommy, why are you crying?"

"Honey, we had to have Rags put to sleep. He was so sick that the doctor couldn't save him."

"Ha—*ha*—ha," he sang and danced around the kitchen floor.

"Tim, do you realize what happened?" his dad questioned.

"My dog died. I don't care. Ha—ha—ha. I'm glad."

I was shaking with a mixture of disbelief and grief. I didn't know what to do or say to him. Kevin was upset and lashed out at Tim. Realizing how disturbed Kevin was, I took him by the hand and led him upstairs to the bedroom.

Ron stayed and tried to talk to Tim. Completely oblivious, he jumped around the room acting silly and singing. "My dog is dead. Ha-Ha. My dog is dead. I don't care. I'm glad."

Tim's response shook us deeply. We wondered why he had laughed. Did he feel any sadness, or was this his strange way of expressing grief? As the days passed Tim never showed any outward signs of grief, nor did he say anything about the loss of his dog.

4

Doctors, Decisions, and Diagnosis

Christmas preparations, along with sorting and packing, pushed the disturbing dog incident out of our minds. Boxes and more boxes were packed and stacked everywhere. We tried to dress our living room for Christmas with festive decorations, but the tree, trimmings, and stacked cartons were a comical conglomeration.

Grandparents, uncles, aunts, and cousins gathered together on Christmas Eve. Grandpa read from the Bible about the Babe in Bethlehem whose birth we celebrated. He reminded us that the Lord had given us the gift we'd prayed for, a home of our own.

We collected a crew of friends and relatives to help us move and by New Year's Eve we were settled. The utility companies were closed for the holiday, so we shivered as we welcomed in the New Year without heat.

The walls of our new home hadn't been painted in at least ten years. They were hideous shades of mustard, turquoise, rose, and dark blue.

The water heater seeped, sizzled, and spewed. Sighing

under the strain of old age, it gasped its final breath and died. In our first month we were properly initiated. We laid the old water heater to rest, installed a new one, and painted the walls.

Kevin and Tim enjoyed their new school. In spring, Tim's kindergarten class incubated eggs. Daily Tim announced how long it would be before the eggs hatched. At open house Tim proudly showed us the new baby chicks.

Tim, however, established a paradoxical pattern between home and school that continued, with one exception, until he was ten years old. At school he showed no signs of his impulsive, unpredictable behavior or his tantrums. He waited until he arrived home from school to explode his bottled frustrations.

From day to day I never knew what to expect. His moods changed unpredictably. Some days he'd arrive home cheerful and played happily like any other rough-and-tumble boy his age. Other days he'd arrive home irritated. Impulsively, he'd dash from one thing to the next, leaving a path of destruction behind.

His rages occurred in unpredictable cycles—sometimes several times a week, other times once a week, or one every two weeks—rarely a month went by without one. Their intensity ranged from an "I-want-my-way!" tantrum to wrath so violent we had to restrain him by clamping our arms and legs around him to prevent him from harming himself or anyone else within reach. Or, if we weren't the target of his anger, he'd try to demolish his room, breaking, smashing, and tearing anything he could grab.

The times when his rages weren't as intense, but he was in an excitable mood, he'd bash a toy or any other item to bits. He loved to climb, but during these times he had no sense of danger. He'd dance and scream senselessly from the roof of our house, or he'd jump off it.

Yet our personal conferences with his kindergarten teachers were positive. We were baffled. Why was he so normal and delightful for several hours or even a stretch of several days? Why did he unexpectedly turn to impulsive destructive behavior and rages with no apparent reason?

At the close of the school year, Tim's report card read, "Tim enjoys all activities of the kindergarten program. He makes good use of his time and takes pride in his work." He was promoted to first grade.

Summer swept us into our usual trips to the beach, parks, and local swimming pools. In the far corner of our yard, partially hidden by the apricot trees, the boys dug a new mudhole, built forts, and made hideouts.

A toothless Tim with a toothless grin tromped off to first grade. I introduced myself to his teacher, Miss Foster. She was plump and not much taller than her first-graders. She had smiling blue eyes, rosy cheeks that glowed, and a vibrant personality. Her classroom was decorated to capture the interest of children. She provided pets to look at and feel, and games to play with during free time. I knew her class would be an exciting place in which to learn.

Kevin and Tim reacted differently to school. Kevin was transferred to a third-fourth combination class. He was placed with the upper grade children in an advanced program. Although he was capable socially, the older children were more mature, which was a bit overwhelming at first.

In the morning Tim aimlessly frittered his time away. He darted from one activity to another. He didn't concentrate on dressing himself or eating breakfast. He harassed Kevin verbally. The longer school day tired Tim. He arrived home starving, crabby, and keyed up.

Ironically, Tim loved his teacher and school. He described the cute dresses she wore. He told us in remarkable detail everything Miss Foster did. If she said something, it was law. If Mom or Dad had anything to say on the same subject, well that was a matter of question.

One situation concerned us. It involved Tim and a boy in his class. His nickname was Hoss, after the Bonanza television character. Hoss was short and stocky, and had an enormous appetite.

One afternoon I talked to Miss Foster. "Tim is having a rough time. He's so irritable after school. How is he doing in class?"

"He's fine except for one thing," she answered. "His friend Hoss has been sneaking part of his lunch. This upsets Tim. I talked with Hoss. I'm sure it won't happen again."

Within a few days, however, Miss Foster called. "I thought you'd like to know that Tim is giving part of his lunch to Hoss."

When I hung up, Tim sensed that it was Miss Foster who called. "Was that my teacher on the phone?"

"Yes, it was. She said that you're giving some of your lunch to Hoss. How come?"

A guilty grin spread across his face. "He's hungry, Mom. He asks me for it."

"Tim, you need your lunch. You come home tired and grumpy because you don't get enough to eat. You can't keep giving your lunch to Hoss."

"But he gets so hungry. He begs me. I feel sorry for him, Mom."

"Your teacher said she'd talk to Hoss's mother. I'm sure he'll bring more food from now on. I know you're worried about Hoss, but you can't feed him anymore."

"Okay, I won't," he finally promised.

In mid-November a parent-teacher-child conference was set for the first school report.

"Tim tries very hard to do his best," Miss Foster smiled. "He's progressing well and is developing good reading habits." She turned to Tim. "You need practice on your handwriting at home. I'm sure your dad and mom will help you. There is one thing we need to solve. Do you think you know what it is?"

"What?" Tim asked, surprised.

"You still give part of your lunch to Hoss."

Sheepishly he smiled. "But I feel sorry for him."

Feeding Hoss was both humorous and frustrating. Failing to convince Tim that Hoss didn't need his food, I decided to practice the old cliché, "When you can't win—join them." Every day I packed extra food for Hoss.

It was a relief. Now Tim will be less tense, I thought. Tim's before-breakfast and after-school impulsiveness, agitated hyperactivity, and tantrums, however, continued unchecked. Concern coupled with constant questioning had grown. "What should we do?" Ron and I asked each other. The certainty that something was wrong and the uncertainty as to what it could be possessed us. Our wait-and-see days were past.

The inner incriminations that maybe we were to blame and had failed as parents haunted us. Should we have listened to the advice of family and friends? "Just a good hard spanking will straighten him up." "He gets too much attention." "You let him have his own way." "He's spoiled!"

We somehow sensed that Tim was not the controller of these odd actions and angry outbursts, but the victim of them. Neither how we reacted nor what we did made any difference in stopping his rage. For several days or only a few hours Tim radiated a static-like electric warning. Then, as if hidden electric current inside Tim was accidentally tripped to high voltage, he'd become increasingly agitated and ignite into an uncontrollable fury. Prior to or following a rage, he'd wander in erratic circles or pace back and forth in a dazed state.

If we remained calm, bodily restrained him, and prevented him from being destructive, the rage didn't last as long. If, however, Ron or I spanked Tim or lashed out verbally, we fanned a fire of wrath that lasted nearly two hours. Like an overloaded circuit which blows a fuse and shuts off all power, Tim crumpled into a soaked, exhausted, starving heap when it was all over.

For Kevin life became trying and difficult. We expected him to be an adult while yet a child. We constantly demanded: "Kevin, control yourself." "Don't make your brother mad." "Leave him alone." "Stop teasing." Kevin rightfully resented bearing the burden of responsibility for Tim's behavior. Our attempts to control Kevin and ourselves in order not to set Tim off were futile.

This wondering and uncertainty became so agonizing that we believed we would welcome any answer. Ron and I agreed to consult Dr. Baldwin, a pediatrician who specialized in the care of children with neurological disorders. When we called to make an appointment, we found that the first available opening was January 29, two months away.

December skidded quickly out of sight and the new year slid in. The afternoon of our visit to Dr. Baldwin finally arrived. Tim and I were nervous as we waited to meet him. The room was small. I squirmed back and forth, unable to make myself comfortable.

Tim sat across from me on a high table, with his legs dangling over the side. I tried to interest him in a toy, but he became distracted by the blood pressure gauge, cotton tips, diaper dispenser, and other paraphernalia.

"Hi, John," the doctor snapped as he entered the room. He was slight of build and short, with a wiry head of salt and pepper hair, a narrow face, and a straight prominent nose.

Tim looked at me and didn't answer.

"Hi, John. How are you today?" The doctor reached out and shook Tim's hand vigorously.

Tim remained silent and pleaded at me with his eyes.

Upset that the doctor didn't know his name, I announced, "His name is not John. His name is Tim."

Dr. Baldwin turned toward me. "I know!" he shot back. "I wanted to see what his response would be."

He opened his folder and took out a five-page form that we'd previously filled out. He asked questions about every phase of my pregnancy, Tim's birth, and his subsequent difficulties and development.

Then he gave Tim a complete physical and had him perform certain motor skill tasks. Dr. Baldwin talked to Tim constantly, asking him questions, giving him commands to test his reflexes, and checking his responses to see if Tim understood what he was saying.

Tim was fidgety. The long process wound him up. Dr. Baldwin completed the exam by telling me, "The history and motor skill test indicate that Tim is hyperkinetic.

"I'm going to give you samples of two types of drugs for him to take. This one will help Tim control himself. He will be able to concentrate better on his schoolwork. This one will help his self-image. He will take one of each in the morning, and one of each before noon at school, and this one when he arrives home. He'll need a blood test, so please stop at the lab on your way out. Bring Tim back in two weeks and I'll see how he is doing."

"Please don't let them give me a shot," Tim begged.

"I'm sorry, honey. It will only take a few seconds."

"Please, Mom, please. I don't want a shot."

We stood at the open door of the lab and the technician asked Tim to sit down. He began to fuss, but the quiet-spoken oriental man tried to soothe him. "It's just like a little bee sting."

He wrapped the rubber tubing around Tim's upper arm and put the needle in his vein. As he did, Tim turned sheet white and passed out.

My heart raced as I saw him slump over. The technician grabbed some ammonia capsules and waved them under Tim's nose. I bent down, wrapped my arms around Tim, and helped him to the car.

My own legs gave way. I was weak and washed out from the ordeal. Tim was distraught and wound up. I tried to soothe him as I drove home.

At first there was no apparent evidence that the drugs were helping Tim gain self-control. At our two-week visit the doctor asked more questions and assured me that it would take time for Tim to adjust to the dosage. He scheduled us for another appointment in three weeks.

Disturbing effects from the drugs appeared. Tim became hazy, lethargic, and glassy-eyed, yet his tantrums continued unchecked. After two weeks of Tim's tyranny and disorientation we decided to try to reach the doctor.

We called Dr. Baldwin and discussed what had happened with Tim. He readjusted the dosage and explained that it would take about a month to six weeks for the drugs to become fully effective. He set an hour-long conference for Ron and me on the second of April so we could discuss Tim's situation further.

It was the early evening supper hour when we arrived at Dr. Baldwin's office. He shook Ron's hand as we entered his study and asked us, "How are things going?" Then he questioned us at length about specific details.

Our discussion centered around the fact that despite Tim's taking two drugs, his tantrums continued. Dr. Baldwin then advised, "I do think that Tim should have an electroencephalogram (EEG). In many cases, uncontrollable rage indicates more than hyperkinesis. I would like you to consult a psychologist at the child guidance clinic to answer some of your questions about Tim's unusual behavior."

For Tim the awesome world of testing devices had returned. Our attempt to hide our apprehension was feeble. Our attitude reflected anxiety and we were unable to explain confidently to Tim why the EEG was essential. This lack of assurance only compounded Tim's confusion and increased his fears.

For the test, Tim could only have six hours sleep. Trying to keep any six-year-old awake, particularly one whose tolerance level is zero, is not easy. It became an endurance contest for the entire family, with long walks, television viewing, and a bath early in the morning to wake Tim up and keep him awake. Our silent prayers sustained us during this stay-awake ordeal.

The test was scheduled for two-thirty in the afternoon. Tim and I left early for Dr. Watkins' office because it was a long drive, and I wasn't sure where it was located. Tim was nervous and scared. We hadn't been informed about what was involved in having an EEG and Tim kept asking questions I couldn't answer. "What are they going to do to me? Will it hurt?"

The waiting room was crowded. The office girl handed me preliminary forms to fill out, then informed me that Dr. Watkins expected his fee in advance.

Before I could complete the forms and write out the check, Tim was called in. I hurriedly gathered my things together and stood to go in with him, but I was told that Tim would have to take the test alone. An expression of fear crossed Tim's face, but he went without protesting.

I had no idea how long the test would take. Aimlessly I thumbed through magazines, but all I could think about was Tim. Time ticked eternally, painfully slow. Although only an hour and a half passed, it seemed like three.

Finally, the nurse came out and told me she needed more information. She eyed me guardedly. I looked dirctly into her eyes while she questioned me and sensed that something was seriously wrong and that she was trying not to let me know.

I asked her if we would be seeing Dr. Watkins next, and would he give us the EEG results. She said she couldn't tell me anything, that Dr. Baldwin would give us the outcome. Then she closed the conversation by telling me Tim would be out in a few minutes.

Tim was tired; his shoulders slumped. He shuffled his feet. I wrapped my arm around him to give him extra support while he walked. I glanced down at his hair and noticed it was matted with sticky white patches of glue.

"They put needles in my brain," Tim complained. "It hurt. They tried to make me sleep, but I didn't want to. My head itches!" On the way home Tim tried to peel off the patches, and small wisps of hair pulled out with the glue. He scratched his head with his fingers, rubbed behind his ears, and tugged on his earlobes.

Prior to the test he'd been too upset to eat all of his lunch. Tim was completely unnerved, irritable, and starved. When we got home, Tim ate a snack, then fell asleep on his bed. I roused him for supper, but he was too tired to eat much, to take a bath, or to have his hair washed. He wanted more than anything to sleep. Ron and I undressed Tim and tucked him into bed. It had been a long night and day. All of us were emotionally and physically drained.

It was April 22 when I took Tim for his checkup and to learn the outcome of the EEG test. The doctor informed me, "The EEG shows that Tim has minimal brain dysfunction and epileptic wave patterns."

"Do you know what caused this to happen?" I asked.

"The mucous plug that delayed his breathing at birth and the resulting lack of oxygen possibly could have caused it. A family history of seizures or epilepsy will sometimes be a factor. He will need an anti-convulsant drug to help him control his outbursts."

"Should he quit taking the two for hyperactivity?"

"No. He needs to take all three because each one meets a specific need or is effective for certain behavior. I want you to come back again in three weeks, and then I'll check him every six weeks after that. If you have any questions before then, be sure to contact me," Dr. Baldwin concluded.

In May we consulted the psychologist, who talked to Tim and then had him draw some pictures. Tim drew pictures of a sunny day and a giraffe grazing in the field. The psychologist assured Ron and me that we were doing everything we could and that the anti-convulsant drug would make a difference.

Looking back on the consultations and the doctor's verdict, I know that Ron and I tried honestly to evaluate our situation.

We wanted help for Tim and ourselves, but we never dreamed it would include all of this.

I don't know when worry moved in and rented a permanent dwelling place, but it did. The financial drain of medical bills and the staggering cost of drugs pushed our budget past its limit. The stress on Ron as provider pressed heavily upon him.

We struggled emotionally with the overwhelming perplexities involved in the high dosage of drugs Tim had to take, our financial situation, our strained family relationships, and the question that pervaded our thoughts most. *What effect does all this have on Tim?*

5

No More Drugs

As the months marched by, Tim relaxed. Anxiety lines that creased his face softened. The seeds of self-confidence started to bloom and his angry outbursts subsided.

The academic pressure of learning the fundamentals of reading, spelling, math, and deciphering simple directions, however, was too much for Tim. By the end of the school year he was considerably behind. We asked Mr. Webster, the principal, if he would allow Tim to repeat the first grade. He denied our request and promoted Tim anyway.

Tim welcomed vacation warmly. He cherished swimming at the beach, exploring parks, our excursion to the San Diego zoo, and wallowing in his mudhole. He sloshed summer into September and was ecstatic his first day of second grade. His next-door friend, Bob, and he were in the same room. A week later he came home crestfallen. Tim had been moved to another room. After six weeks, two rooms, and three teachers he was settled for the year.

His teacher was slender, with waist-length dark brown hair. She had the contrasting qualities of firmness and warmth—a direct manner of speaking and a delightful sense of humor. She radiated a sense of security to which Tim responded well.

In January we received Tim's report card. The A-B-C grading system had been dropped. It was impossible to tell accurately how he was doing, except for the fact that his reading level was at the first grade, seventh-month level. He was behind almost one year. The teacher's comment on his card read:

> Tim's poor work habits and short interest span hamper his reading ability. I find that when you are able to help him at home with his word list and spelling words, he does much better. Tim does quite well in the area of mathematics, but would be helped greatly if he could gain speed in computing number facts. He enjoys classroom participation and has many good ideas and interesting suggestions to share with the class.

In mid-March Tim complained that he was dizzy, lightheaded, having headaches, and seeing spots. There were times when he was afraid the floor would hit him in the face, and he nodded off to sleep in school. Although the drugs were not supposed to be habit-forming, Ron and I struggled with Tim's need to take three different drugs, a total of nine pills a day.

Dr. Baldwin had an extremely busy practice. During our frequently interrupted, in-and-out sessions we weren't given adequate time to describe Tim's condition.

Finally during an office visit toward the end of March I persisted in describing Tim's disoriented state of being. Dr. Baldwin suspected Tim was experiencing an adverse drug reaction. He temporarily removed two of the drugs Tim was taking, ordered a series of blood tests, and another EEG for April. By the time Tim and I reached the lab, Tim was extremely upset and passed out when the technician took the blood sample.

On the way home he pleaded, "Please don't let them do the brain wave thing again."

During the next few days his dad and I tried to explain to Tim why he had to have another EEG. Yet we both cringed at the thought of his being subjected to the test again. Ron adamantly promised, "Tim, we'll never make you have another one—ever again!"

Ron and I prayed for Tim more fervently than we had ever prayed before. We asked our family and friends to pray with us that Tim would be well and able to function normally without drugs.

Since Tim could only have six hours sleep before the test, we let him choose something special to pass the time away. A double-feature Charlie Brown movie was showing and Tim wanted to see it. Both boys and I sat through the two features, but it was only 10 P.M. when it was over.

"Let's sit through it once more," I suggested. Tim, however, started falling asleep.

"Wake up. Wake up. You can't sleep."

"I'm so tired. Please let me sleep," he mumbled.

"You can't sleep. You'll ruin the test. Come on," I shook him, but he still dozed off. "Let's get up and walk."

Tim lurched up the aisle, then staggered out into the lobby like a drunk. I held on to him to keep him on his feet. The glaring stares of the theater personnel and patrons told us that he was up too late.

We drove to a local restaurant where Tim and Kevin ordered a treat. The staying-up goal was 12:30 A.M. It was now only 11:30.

We still had a half hour left when we arrived home. We turned on midnight television, which is not the most child-oriented. Tim was so exhausted that he could hardly focus his eyes on the screen. I stood him on his feet and tried to walk him around, but he slept as he walked. Finally I put Tim to bed. Ron agreed to rise earlier than usual in the morning to wake Tim.

The test was scheduled for 9:30 A.M. Tim and I were weary and hardly spoke as we drove to Dr. Watkins' office. In the reception room I leaned back to rest. I prayed that Tim would never have to endure this test again. Would his progress be permanent? I prayed so. Would his overdosed drug world soon come to an end? I hoped so.

Two weeks later on April 14, exactly a year from Tim's previous EEG, Dr. Baldwin revealed the results. He examined the report carefully, and then smiled. "The test came out completely clear. There is no sign of abnormal brain waves."

"We've kept Tim off the two drugs, even though he was to resume taking them after the EEG," I stammered. "He's been fine. His teacher reports he isn't falling asleep in class. Should we keep him on the one drug he's continued to take?"

"Yes, and keep him off the other medication for a while. We'll see how he does. We'll check him in two months."

Ron and I were jubilant. Our prayers were being answered. Tim was pleased. Now he would no longer need to feel embarrassed by taking pills at school.

In May, Tim complained again that he was dizzy and still seeing spots. This time the doctor took him off the last drug to see if he was having a reaction to it.

We were overjoyed. No more drugs! We called our friends and family to tell them that Tim was free—free from drugs. Our confidence was growing that he was finally well.

The last week of school Tim received a certificate of award for "Special Overall Improvement" in the all-school assembly.

When Tim came home the last day of school, he brought along his final report card. We read it over together. He received equal amounts of *most of the times* and *some of the times* and didn't have any *not yets*.

All we could do was guess that his report was average, considering he didn't receive any *not yets*. (*Not yet what?* I wondered.) What his teacher had to say made more sense and encouraged us:

> Tim has worked hard since last report and is doing very well in math. He has begun to master the skills of renaming and multiplication and I'm very proud of him! Tim has worked very hard this year and I know he's earned this summer break. I've enjoyed watching his

progress and hope he'll continue the good work.

When we reached the bottom of the report Tim moaned, "Oh, no. I have Cindy's teacher, Mrs. Ellerby, next year. She yells at the kids."

"How do you know?" I asked. "The card only says room thirty-two."

"I know, I know. That's where Cindy is now."

"Just because Mrs. Ellerby has that room this year doesn't mean she'll have it next year."

Cindy's mother and I had chuckled over Mrs. Ellerby's hot-tempered ways. She was from the old school that demanded no-nonsense discipline. She had a reputation for shaping kids up and sending them off to fourth-grade better students. Cindy was spirited, high-strung, and listening wasn't her best subject. Her mom agreed that Mrs. Ellerby had settled her down. She might be just the teacher Tim needs, I thought. On the other hand, I wondered.

Walt and Shirley Taylor, our church family friends, invited the boys and me to go with them to Hume Lake Camp. Dale, their oldest son, and Kevin would be in wagon train junior camp. Tim and I would stay in a cabin with Walt, Shirley, and their youngest son, David. The tranquillity that a Christian camp atmosphere provides would be a welcome rest.

Cradled together since infancy in our church nursery, Sunday School, and our homes, the four boys had formed a friendship closer than most brothers. Tim and David—a tousle-haired blond with snapping brown eyes—had developed an even closer, almost radar twin-like closeness. David's loving ways, wisdom, and calm manner of approaching life soothed Tim.

David and Tim gathered treasures for the trip. They bought candy, collected odds and ends of precious toys, and haggled over items they were sure they couldn't survive without. Finally we set a limit. We were cramming seven people, food, and gear for a week at camp in one station wagon.

Like a nest sitting on the top branches of a tree, Hume Lake Camp nestles on the crest of the Sequoia National Forest. In the distant horizon the pines that line the lake look like a handful of fingers caressing the powder blue sky. A brilliant freshness, peace, and indescribable beauty graces this retreat.

When we reached the entrance, buses were unloading young people. The din of happy voices shouting greetings to friends punctuated the air.

We climbed the hill to register and joined the chattering band of campers. First we checked into our cabin, then delivered Dale and Kevin, who were eager to explore their covered wagon campgrounds.

That week we trudged over the hills, hiked behind the lake, crawled on slippery rocks in the waterfall, basked in the warm sun, and perched on mammoth rocks in the early morning to renew our relationship with our Lord.

Tim and David spent every available minute wading in the lake and stream. They searched for huge tadpoles and frogs, which they scooped up and captured with old cans and foam cups.

They trapped hundreds of these creatures. Our cabin porch was decorated with various sizes of pans and cans of tadpoles and frogs. The frogs escaped regularly. The tadpoles died when the water seeped out of leaky cups. The boys tended their captive pets lovingly and mourned when they escaped or died.

We climaxed the week with a fish fry and devotional on Inspiration Mountain high above the lake. It was a week of spiritual refreshment and emotional renewal.

As our sun-bathed summer came to a close we felt more confident and wanted to believe Tim was well. It had been almost five months since he had been on drugs. We convinced ourselves that he was just a highly-active boy and an incurable tease.

Late one August afternoon I was resting on the couch and reading the latest magazine that had just arrived in the mail.

"Help, help! Someone help me," I heard from somewhere

in the distant outside. *Sounds like some kids fooling around.*

"Help, Help! Please, help me," the voice pleaded. Tired, I continued to rest.

"Help, help!" *That's John. I wonder why his mother doesn't check on him. She was just out there.*

A few minutes of quiet and then, "Help, somebody please help me." The caller pleaded a few more times.

I glanced at the clock. Fifteen minutes had passed. Putting down my magazine, I charged out our door and surveyed the neighboring yards. As I started walking toward the front sidewalk, I caught a glimpse of a child hanging by his neck high up in the tree.

My heart thundered in my chest as I raced to see who it was. A flash of horror passed through my mind that I could have let a child hang there so long; how would I ever get him down?

"TIM—Tim are you—"

Interrupting me, he laughed hilariously. "Ha, ha, ha! I fooled you."

He had hung the nape of his shirt on a branch and pretended to dangle from the tree, screaming. He hoped to scare a passerby or gain my attention with his screaming pleas.

"Get down from there! You scared me half to death. Don't you *ever* do that again! It's not funny. Stop laughing. Right now! You could give someone a coronary doing this. Now hurry up and get down." A steady stream of commands poured out of me, expelling my exasperation and fright. "You go to your room and stay there for a while," I ordered, grabbing Tim by the arm and marching him to his room.

6

Road to Regression

When school opened Tim did have Mrs. Ellerby for his third-grade teacher. From the beginning, Tim complained, "Mrs. Ellerby yells so loud she hurts my ears."

Thinking it would help, I explained Tim's past in detail to Mrs. Ellerby. I told her he'd been on drugs but no longer needed them. She had a convincing sureness about her. I rationalized that her strict approach was just the dose of medicine Tim needed. She was sure she could help him and felt strongly that drugs were not the solution.

Kevin, now in the fifth grade, was in a combination fifth-sixth class, and would be doing mostly sixth-grade work. Gray-brown, straight-as-straw hair accented his round face, wide turned-up nose, and sensitive blue eyes. Quiet in disposition, he sought solitude, searching for a place he could call his own.

At home Kevin was usually absorbed in his own activities, masterminding or creating a new project, reading books, or collecting shells, insects, and stamps. His warm sense of humor, unexpected quips, and perception of life always surprised us.

Magic, his current pastime, turned into an all-consuming

hobby for Kevin. He scoured the library shelves for magic books, taught himself the secrets, and practiced hours at a time. One afternoon he announced that he'd like to do magic shows for birthday parties. To advertise his new service, he made posters and cards to put up in local stores.

Halfheartedly I encouraged him. I was engaged in directing a parent-participation nursery school, attending meetings, involved in church activities, and the umpteen other responsibilities of working and taking care of a family. I felt Kevin was too young to start his own business. It would complicate my chaotic schedule and I had no intention of taking him to put up posters or do shows. It never occurred to Ron and me that Kevin would pursue his magic interests as avidly as he did.

It was lunchtime, the first of November. My arms were piled with books, papers, and school paraphernalia. I had just walked in the front door from work when the phone rang. "It's a mother from school," I grumbled to myself, "and I haven't even had time to eat lunch."

Trying to juggle everything, I grabbed the phone. "I read your son's letter in the newspaper and I was interested in knowing more about his magic shows," the caller informed me.

"You read my son's—what? Where?" I exclaimed. My juggling act was off balance and books and papers scattered to the floor.

"Tell me again, *please*," I stammered.

"Your son's letter was in the paper, stating he does magic."

"I didn't know he sent anything in. When did it come out?"

"This morning," the man chuckled.

"Well—aaaa—we get an evening paper. Could you please read it to me?"

Dear Trouble Shooter:

> I am ten years old and I do party magic shows. If you will print my letter in your column, I might get some publicity. I charge five dollars for a show and I supply party favors and prizes.
>
> K.C.

The price sounds fair enough. I admire young people with "get up and go," so I'm going to ask parents whose youngsters have birthday parties coming up soon if they'd be interested in trying out your magic party service. They can address their inquiries to Kevin Cragg, 3870 Oak Street.

"You're right, that's our son. Well, well," I stammered again. "He isn't home from school and I'll have to wait until he gets here to discuss this with him." I tried to patch up my shocked state by mumbling something about the fact that he was good at magic.

I no sooner had hung up when the phone started to ring and ring and ring! What surprised me was that our number wasn't listed in the newspaper. Everyone had looked it up in the phone book. Finally I had to take the phone off the hook until Kevin and his dad arrived home.

When Kevin came in at 3:00 P.M. I inquired, "A man called and said your letter for magic shows appeared in the newspaper. When did you send it in?"

"It did! Where is it?"

"It was in the morning paper. Our paper hasn't come yet. When did you send it in?" I asked again.

"A coupla weeks ago."

"You didn't ask us if you could do this. How come?"

"Well—you wouldn't take me to the store to put up my cards. I got tired of waiting around, so I sent it in. Besides, I need money to buy more magic tricks."

The paper arrived before their dad did, and the boys bombarded him with the news the minute he walked in. Laughing when he read it, Ron congratulated Kevin. "That's great, son. You're turning into a real celebrity."

"I don't think it's funny," I moaned.

Ron had always been a frustrated comedian, and his only audience had been his family. He had entertainment blood in his bones. Since his own father had been a clown, harmonica player, and singer in his youth, Kevin's interest in magic tickled Ron's own secret show business dreams. Immediately they began to plan what Kevin would wear and how he would do his act.

"Now wait a minute," I desperately interrupted. "How will I ever work, go to school nights, keep up the house, and take him to magic shows? You'll have to help too, Ron!"

Ignoring me, they continued to make plans.

"Kevin, where are you going to get those party favors you promised?" I interjected.

"Remember the carnival supply place where you got some nursery school stuff last summer?"

He has all this planned out. That's for sure.

"What about the money to buy them with?" I questioned.

"Could you lend me the money? I'll pay you back when I earn my own."

Fifteen dollars worth of party favors, new black shoes, pants, and top hat later, plus a suit jacket from the Goodwill store, our son, Kevin Cragg—The Little Magic Man—was outfitted. Three shows were booked for the next Saturday and more were scheduled to follow.

Being so wrapped up in directing preschool and Kevin's new career I had ignored Tim's continuing complaints. I had kept reminding myself that he was well now and he'd survive. In the morning he was tense, "My stomach aches. Can I stay home?" After school it was, "I have a headache."

On December 15 we were thrust back into the world of reality. Our first child-parent-teacher conference had been scheduled for this day. Tim brought home a paper with the "Child's Goals" printed on the back. "I am good in drawing, I need extra work in spelling, and My goals are playing," were scrawled in Tim's printing.

During the conference we found that "My goals are playing," was actually meant to be: "My goals are to stop playing in the room." Still no grades, his progress report card read *Is learning* and *Has learned*. The *Is learning* far outnumbered the

Has learned, and he was in a beginning second-grade reading book in the third grade.

"He doesn't pay attention and needs to work faster," Mrs. Ellerby berated Tim. Pensively he sat there, saying nothing. Her unrelenting barrage of words overwhelmed us, and we both sat silently as she complained about Tim. "He's unable to take dictated spelling words or sentences. He can't write stories or do any work unless I personally give him the instructions."

We consulted Dr. Baldwin, who told us to ask Mrs. Ellerby not to pressure Tim or require him to do dictated spelling and stories because he was not able to do them.

Every day Tim poured out his distress. "Mrs. Ellerby blows her top." "She pulls my hair." "She talks too fast." "She screams at me when I don't understand." "She breaks rulers over the desk when she's mad. Yaa—she's nice to your face, Mom, but not to me."

One afternoon he announced, "My teacher threw an eraser at me. I ducked and she missed me," he giggled. "She told me the next time she wouldn't miss."

Although Tim had steadily regressed since a few months after he stopped taking drugs, his tantrums, overactivity, and impulsiveness intensified under this stress. I talked with Mr. Webster, who agreed with my complaints about Mrs. Ellerby's yelling, but somehow he was able to excuse her actions.

As the year progressed Tim dropped farther and farther behind. On March 15, we had a second conference. His teacher wrote on his report, "Tim has difficulty concentrating on his lessons. We will continue working together. He has shown some progress." The report had now been changed to *partial mastery* and *achieved mastery*, of which he seemed to have equal amounts.

In reading, and in some other areas, Tim was a year behind. He still needed individualized directions and couldn't do his spelling or write stories.

I asked Mrs. Ellerby, "Do you think Tim should repeat the third grade?"

"No, I don't think so. He's doing the best he ever will do. It would be best to push him forward."

"But they have a rotating schedule. How will he ever survive?"

"Other kids have problems and they make it through," she replied.

Tim wouldn't walk to the local market four blocks away for fear he'd get lost, and they expected him to find his way to six different classes! Tim couldn't do his work without constant supervision. Would six teachers give him directions? Large-group reading had as many as sixty children in the auditorium at once. How would he survive this? We were in a quandary, unsure what we should do.

Then in April Tim broke for the first time at school. During early recess, he became so enraged at a classmate that he held him to the ground and pounded him with his fists. They had to pry Tim loose and bodily remove him from the playground. Instead of calling Ron or me at work, the principal suspended Tim for the day and sent him to a neighbor.

We knew we had to take action on our own. The local council of the preschool where I worked had a consultant service which offered psychological counseling at a reduced rate. We made an appointment in May with Dr. Caldwell for Tim to take educational tests which would evaluate his abilities.

In our search for solutions, certain questions pursued us. Should we seek a smaller remedial education class, hold Tim back a year, or secure state aid for specialized private schooling? Despite the fact that both Ron and I worked, we were still unable to afford the $100 to $250 monthly tuition that private schooling required.

I went to see the principal again to find out the procedure for seeking the special education and to tell him that Tim would be taking the tests.

Nonchalantly he replied, "First send the results to me and I'll look them over."

I somehow sensed there was more to the procedure than he

expressed. I contacted the local school district office. The district secretary informed me that the cutoff date for the initial report was the last week of school. If I sent or took the reports to the principal for his consideration we could not meet the district deadline and our appeal for educational assistance would be delayed until the next year. As it was, we would have to ask the psychologist to rush his report to the district office.

Mrs. Ellerby knew about the tests, and when Tim came home a few days later his bleak eyes and bewildered expression told me he was upset. When Tim spoke, I observed an anguish beyond anything that had been before.

"My teacher said to me, 'Your parents are wasting all that money on you for nothing! If you'd settle down and do your work, they wouldn't have to do this!' "

Unbelief and shock jolted me. When Ron came home that night I told him what had happened. Nothing would be gained to think again the thoughts Ron and I shared, both spoken and unspeakable. Resentment, disillusionment, and the desire to defend ourselves shadowed our thinking.

This experience confused Tim and depleted his already diminished self-image. Any progress he had made was completely undone by now. The shock of Tim's decline to where he was before he went on drugs haunted us. Yet neither Ron nor I could face Tim's being on drugs again. So we placed the weight of our hopes on changing his school situation.

We encouraged Tim to do his best and try to endure the remaining days of the school year. To lighten his load, we decided that whatever testing or decisions that were made would be our secret. We promised him that we would not tell his teacher or principal anything more. But it would be many years before the trauma Tim endured that year began to heal, and even then it left an indelible mark.

7

Tests, Tests, and More Tests!

When we consulted Dr. Caldwell for the final test results, he confirmed Tim's need for remedial schooling with therapy to help him develop his auditory perception. He asked us to see our pediatrician and have him fill out the additional papers that were required. He set a time for us to consult with Mr. Brower, a speech and hearing specialist, who would also examine Tim and give his professional opinion.

Tim and I went to confer with his pediatrician, Dr. Baldwin. "My, you've lost a lot of weight," Dr. Baldwin told me without asking why Tim and I were there to see him. "You look great. How'd you do it?"

"I've been going to Weight Watchers," I remarked. "I came in today to see if you could help us get Tim into a specialized learning class. Tim has had a rough year and is behind in his schoolwork. Dr. Caldwell did some tests and recommended that we see you."

Dr. Baldwin ignored my statement. "How much weight have you lost?"

"Thirty-six pounds."

"Do you like the Weight Watcher diet? I've put on a little

weight," he patted his stomach. "You look terrific!"

I couldn't bring Dr. Baldwin back to the discussion about Tim's special needs. He casually scanned Tim's March report card, suggested we have Dr. Caldwell send the tests to him, then turned the topic back to me.

Dr. Baldwin's practice had mushroomed; his heavy load pressed him into pushing his patients through quickly. He hadn't taken time to concentrate on Tim's needs. Now his discussion centered on my weight loss! That evening Ron and I debated the situation at length. We concluded that although we knew it would be confusing for Tim we should change doctors.

We contacted Dr. Kenyon, a pediatrician who had been highly recommended and specialized in the care of hyperkinetic children. We were told that he took time to talk to both parents and children, and that he limited his practice to meet his patients' needs. We set an appointment for June 5.

Dr. Kenyon was a tall, jovial, heavyset man with wavy blond-brown hair. His manner was relaxed and direct. Tim, however, was panic-stricken. He was sure that he would have to have another EEG and more blood tests.

As Dr. Kenyon proceeded with the preliminary checkup, he promised Tim that he would not have to have either a shot or an EEG. He had Tim perform motor skill tasks and gave him a complete physical. He read over the reports of the psychologist, talked to us at length, and concurred that Tim needed specialized schooling.

School ended the second week of June and the closing comments on Tim's report card read:

> Does not always listen. Tim has improved. Has health problems which contribute to frustration in certain areas, which has been discussed.
>
> September placement: *Grade four.*

I kept in close contact with the school district office. On Wednesday of the week school was out, I phoned Mr. Walker, who was handling our case.

"I'm sorry, Mrs. Cragg, but we can't accept Dr. Caldwell's

findings, or the speech and hearing tests. We feel Dr. Caldwell slanted his report to suit the results he desired. According to the IQ test we gave, and the reports in Tim's file, we don't think Dr. Caldwell is correct."

"But you took those tests when Tim was in first grade. You've never seen Tim since then."

"We do not recognize Dr. Caldwell," he firmly stated. Then went on to explain why he personally didn't like him. I was too stunned to remember everything he said.

"Well, then, what about Dr. Kenyon's report?" I asked.

"Didn't you say that Dr. Baldwin was your son's doctor?"

"Yes, at one time, but we changed."

"The only doctor we recognize is Dr. Baldwin. He's a well-known authority. His reputation is established across the nation. We prefer working with him. I don't even know Dr. Kenyon. I'm sorry, but we won't do anything unless we hear from Dr. Baldwin."

"Why didn't you tell us this in the first place? You knew whom we were consulting," I retorted.

I was too dazed to hear his reply or answer back. I kept thinking, "The future of a child is at stake, not someone's reputation."

Ron and I discussed the dilemma in which we now found ourselves. We knew our only alternative was to see Dr. Baldwin again. We felt trapped in what seemed an overpowering game of politics. We wondered if we'd ever find help because our son needed it, not because we knew the right person who owned the right key.

The last week of June, Kevin and Tim were to go to Hume Lake Camp with the Taylors. Earlier in the year Walt and Shirley had added a new member to their household, and she would be going to camp, too. Teresa was in their home under the county foster care program. She was a brown-eyed, two-year-old Mexican-American beauty, with a spunky, independent, and charming personality.

When she arrived, Tim was fascinated by her and concerned that she would be happy in her new home.

One day, shortly after she came to the Taylors, he strolled out of his room with something hidden behind his back. "Mom, can we go see Teresa?" he asked. "I want to give her this to keep her company." He giggled self-consciously, then brought out his battered, beloved, turquoise teddy bear.

"Can we go right now?"

"Yes, we sure can," I answered, surprised.

When we entered the Taylors' house, Tim bent down on his knees and awkwardly thrust his teddy bear in front of Teresa. He grinned and patted her. "Here, Teresa. Here, Teresa. This is for you."

She backed away because she was still shy in her new surroundings. It touched me to see Tim give his treasured teddy bear away.

At camp Tim, David, and Teresa stayed in a cabin with the Taylors. Dale and Kevin were in Wagon Train Junior Camp.

The week the boys were gone was a welcome rest. Ron and I had time alone together to think things through, renew our own relationship, and to sort out our battered feelings.

On Friday, we received a concise camp letter handwritten by Tim.

> Tim Cragg
>
> Dear mom and dad I miss you we were by a squirrel. we caught a big pollywagg I found a knife we wint boat ridding we saw baby fishs we got a hide out we fed the horses we saw a deer we have a five leaf clover

Two days after camp, on Monday, July 3, we went to see Dr. Baldwin. Knowing Tim had already endured enough, I left Kevin and him in the waiting room and went in to see the doctor by myself.

I was totally preoccupied with our predicament. I couldn't tell Dr. Baldwin that we were going to take Tim to a different pediatrician, and yet I would have to tell him about the psychologist's reports the school district had rejected.

It would be an understatement to say that I had no inkling, nor could ever have predicted what was to happen in the doctor's office that day.

When Dr. Baldwin entered the small examination room, I was sitting on a bench in a cubbyhole corner. Before I could speak he exclaimed, "You look terrific! How much more weight have you lost?"

A bit embarrassed I tried to change the subject and talk to him about Tim. He ignored my questions and continued his praises. He started walking toward me and as he bent down I realized what he was going to do. I was trapped with no way to escape. I turned my head and pulled away, hitting the wall.

He grabbed my cheeks between his hands and planted a kiss on my fleeting face.

"I was only trying to show you how great you look." He backed off as if surveying a prize he'd just won and captured. His face was red, his breathing heavy. He was obviously shaken. So was I!

Panic set in, and I started praying, "God, help me get out of here!"

Abruptly he announced that he had a telephone call he had to answer in the next room (no one had paged him), and he turned and left the room.

Stunned, I couldn't decide which to do first, flee or scream. He reentered the room almost immediately.

I quickly chose a cold, calculating, straightforward approach and took complete command of the conversation. I almost ordered him to read the reports.

Still dazzled, he hadn't recuperated and couldn't read the report or concentrate on my conversation. Finally he suggested that we take Tim to a well-known speech and hearing center.

I stood to my feet and continued talking a mile-a-minute as I edged my way around him and opened the door to leave. Like a doctor giving orders to his patient, I repeated the same sentence several times, asking him to write the school district to help Tim get special schooling.

His fleeting remark was: "You know I'd do *anything* to help you." (Help me? I'm sure!)

When I told Ron, he was sober at first and then he broke into laughter.

Indignant and insulted, I demanded, "What's so funny? I certainly don't see any humor in this!"

Through peals of laughter he gasped out that when he pictured this five-foot, one-inch, wiry, skinny, doctor making a pass at his five-foot, seven-and-a-half-inch wife, he couldn't help laughing.

"I don't think it's funny at all," I retorted. But when I pictured the incident again, through his eyes, I began giggling. It was the only relief we had from the ridiculous predicament we were in. Despite the fact that Dr. Baldwin was our key to special education, this incident clinched our decision never to return to his office again.

The speech and hearing clinic told us they had an appointment that had been canceled, on July 5, two days away. Tim could come at that time; otherwise he would have to wait until late August. We still had district deadlines to meet and accepted the appointment, even though that was the day we had planned to leave on our family vacation.

The morning of the fifth, Tim woke early, eagerly anticipating our trip and yet apprehensive at being confronted again with this constant questioning.

The clinic consisted of several reconverted older homes which had been made into a preschool, testing center, and therapy rooms. The parkway between the sidewalk and street was lined with immense trees.

We checked with the receptionist, who asked us to be seated while she notified the speech therapist of our arrival. Within a few minutes the therapist joined us, introduced herself, and asked us to follow her.

She ushered me into another waiting room filled with parents, children, and babies waiting to be called on for speech therapy. She informed me that the test would take an hour, after which she would have a conference with me. The time passed quickly and I was surprised when the therapist returned with Tim.

She told Tim he could go outside to play. I bid him a quick good-bye and followed her down another long hallway and into a small room. We sat across the table from each other. Quietly she read over the test, not speaking a word to me.

These consultations and constant scrutiny were not easy. I wondered what opinions they formed about me, our family, and Tim. Would they help me unravel a small piece of this tangled thread that bound us so tightly? Would we gain any new insights this time? What did they write about us in their reports?

We knew these tests would be in Tim's permanent school records and that they would follow him through high school into adulthood. We could only hope that these professionals would not use their power to misjudge us.

The possibility of these reports having lifelong effects on Tim and following him, pegging him, and placing him in a box that he could not break out of weighed heavily upon us. Would our intentions to help him turn on us so that we wished we had never subjected him to all this?

The therapist straightened the papers in front of her and then began talking. "I cannot calculate the total results yet, but I will show you what I have completed. Tim sees pictures as fragments and not as a whole. He is weakest in auditory perception, short-term and sequential memory, visual association, and associating family groupings. He doesn't understand the concepts of change and plurality in words such as good-better-best. He excels in manual dexterity and verbal expression."

Wild and emotionally pent-up, Tim climbed the outside wall of the house, peeked over the windowsill, and asked repeatedly, "What are you doing? I want to go home."

Finally after we repeatedly told him that if he let us talk we could leave sooner, he left us alone and we were able to go on.

"He is *very upset*!" she stated. "He was over-anxious and worried when I worked with him." She eyed me almost accusingly. "He thinks you're unhappy with him and that he can't do anything right. He wonders what is wrong with him."

I was aggravated, grieved, and I knew I could not divulge the political problems nor my encounter with Dr. Baldwin. All I could do was try to clarify her statement by explaining.

"You're the *sixth* person either to examine or test Tim since May, and this is the second time he's taken this test. I realize what this is doing to him and it upsets me. This testing has been more destructive to him than some of his problems!"

"Then that's why he was so familiar with parts of the test," she replied. "As you know," she continued without questioning me further, "Tim is nine years, one month, at this time. His scores range from the six-year and six-month level to nine years and ten months. The majority of the scores are below eight years and one month, with only two scores at the level of nine years."

She leafed through the papers showing me more of the scores. "The results of this test are identical to the one he took in May," I interjected. "Do you have any suggestions as to how we can help him?"

"He needs help in the area of short-term memory. Assign him a task, like setting the table; then give him simple directions. Start with no more than two or three steps to a task. When he can do that, increase the number of instructions.

"Ask him to repeat them to you to see if he understands. Make sure he carries the work out in sequence. Go over the directions again if you need to. Gradually give him more complicated tasks. This is a simple way you can help him at home. He will need special education to help him in other areas," she concluded.

I was hungry, tired, and my head ached and pounded rhythmically. When I found Tim he was perched in the top of a tree near the car.

As we drove along. Tim shared what had gone on while I

talked to the speech therapist. He complained, "I'm hungry and my head hurts." Then he confessed, "A lady came to get me down out of the tree. '*Get down from there*,' she said. '*No*,' I told her. She told me to get down again, but I told her, '*No*.'

" '*What's your name*?' she asked me. '*Batman*,' I said. She asked me again and I told her, '*Batman*.'

"When I got down she grabbed me by the arm. I pushed her and hit her. She was so scared of me her hands shook."

"Oh, no, Tim," I sighed.

Anxiety creased his eyes, but he continued to talk in his own frantic way. "She sat me on a chair and asked the lady at the desk my name. She told her Tim Cragg. I jerked my arm away and ran out of there. I climbed the fence and got back up in the tree. She didn't bother me anymore."

Tim was famished, overwhelmed, and devastated. By the time we completed our half-hour drive, we were both exhausted and hardly in the mood to leave for a long trip to Big Bear Lake.

Throughout our vacation and after we arrived home, the prevailing question Ron and I discussed was whether I should quit teaching preschool. Directing preschool had been the creative highlight of my life. It gave me the opportunity to express myself in ways which were meaningful to me. Yet I knew Tim needed more attention than I was able to give when working.

God's steady, still small voice haunted me with the conviction that what I loved so much had to be set aside. It was only after I had written my letter of resignation in late July that I had assurance and peace that I had made the right decision.

8

Smile, God Loves You

For close to ten years our little white church had been the sanctuary where we shared our personal triumphs and griefs and received affirmation and compassion in return. Like a skillful weaver, Christ in His love had woven us into His spiritual Body.

Our chapel was nestled between green hibiscus and a peaceful olive tree. Nearby was a sprawling pepper tree to climb, hideouts, a canal with fish, toads in the shrubs, and a school play yard. Our children's classes were creative, flexible, and adapted to a practical living faith. It was Tim's second home.

After church one Sunday evening Tim called his dad into his room. "Daddy, I want to accept Christ." Ron shared with him and together they prayed a prayer confessing Christ as Saviour and Lord.

When Pastor Lloyd invited young people and children to join a new believers' class, Tim wanted to attend. We were concerned the study book might be too difficult for him, but when Tim didn't understand he'd ask Pastor Lloyd to explain. Over the next weeks Tim's understanding grew. We watched him embrace Christ's love, and an observable change quietly took place in his attitude.

September rested on August's threshold and still the school district had not confirmed where Tim would be placed. The transition from vacation to school and school to vacation normally upset Tim. The anticipation prior to a change, the broken routines during a change, and not knowing what to expect increased the tension and set him off.

Finally, the school district made its decision. They refused to place Tim in a special class or sign for state funds for private school. Despite his disabilities, the test, and doctor reports, Tim didn't qualify. The district psychologist said that Tim should repeat third grade and wondered why he hadn't been kept back earlier. We were given the choice of allowing Tim to return to his former school or transferring him to another school three blocks away. We chose to have him transferred to the new school because they did not have the rotating junior high-type classes.

"Please don't make me go," Tim begged, obviously distraught. "I won't have any friends. What if my teacher gets mad at me?"

I was depressed and felt forsaken. Had God abandoned us? "Why, God, why?" I questioned. "Why has all this happened?" We felt we had no real choice. We could not afford private schooling. Despite my despair, God's seeming silence only existed in my mind.

I called for an appointment with Mrs. Johnson, the principal. She set a time for me to see her the following Friday, only a week before school was to open. She was a tall, well-dressed woman with auburn hair, a broad face, and a warm smile.

My prayer of desperation had been that God would help the principal understand Tim's problem and give him the teacher he needed. As our conversation progressed, God's presence calmed my inner anxieties. Mrs. Johnson explained, "I've worked closely with hyperkinetic children. We have a learning disability class here at our school and if Tim needs it we can place him there. I will read his records and observe him in the classroom. I have chosen Mrs. Davis, who is a newer teacher. She is positive, patient, and has a special way of working with children. I think you will like her."

"Could I bring Tim in and let him meet you and see his classroom?" I inquired.

"I would like to meet Tim. Come back at two o'clock this afternoon."

I can still remember the summer breeze, and how the sunshine glistened on the elm trees in the parkway as I left her office. My heart rejoiced with thanksgiving as I realized God was answering our prayers.

Tim was scared and restless when I took him to meet Mrs. Johnson. She stood behind the counter, smiling warmly at Tim. Trying to draw Tim out, she asked questions about his summer.

A fretful expression filled his face and shyness suddenly shadowed him. He was unable to respond to her, and instead he looked at me to see if I would answer for him. He fidgeted and rocked from side to side on his feet. Written all over Tim was an overwhelming feeling of futility at being confronted with this new school situation.

After trying unsuccessfully to communicate with Tim, Mrs. Johnson showed him where his room was located, across the hall from her office. Glad to be free, he hurried out of the room.

Before I could leave she asked me, "Is Tim on any medication?"

"No, he hasn't been for almost a year now," I replied.

"I think it would be wise if you asked his doctor to prescribe something for him. He's very nervous. It might help him to concentrate in the classroom."

"Yes, I'm sure he probably does need something. I'll check it out." I had known for a long time that sooner or later Tim would be on drugs again, but it wasn't easy to face.

Ron and I acknowledged that although we knew Tim needed a drug to calm his overactivity, to increase his attention span, and hopefully to prevent his rages, we could not face subjecting him to the disoriented overdosed drug world of the past.

Monday morning! School opened. The sidewalk and lawn were alive with brightly arrayed children modeling their new shoes, pants, dresses, and shirts. The girls twisted, turned, and giggled. The boys pushed, shoved, and shouted. Old acquaintances were being renewed. Apprehensively, Tim got out of the car and quietly joined the crowd.

Tuesday afternoon we had another appointment with Dr. Kenyon. Tim was overwrought.

"Don't let him give me a shot. And I don't want another brain wave," he pleaded over and over.

Reluctantly Tim followed me into the waiting room. When he sat down, he bounced and jiggled up and down. He got up to see the aquarium of fish, then bolted for the door. I was watching him closely and reached the door before he could escape. I pulled him back to the couch and tried to interest him in a magazine. The receptionist, realizing Tim was upset, called us into the inner waiting room.

A musical marching band of men was printed on the wallpaper. I had Tim count the number of men, their instruments, and anything I could think of to occupy his mind.

In his easygoing manner, Dr. Kenyon tried to talk with Tim during the examination. Tim thrashed around. His eyes were vacant. He refused to cooperate.

Being subjected to all this probing devastated Tim and destroyed his already diminished self-image. One time he would strike out in self-defense against an unbearable world. At other times he would strive again and again to achieve a selfhood he could claim with respect.

He wondered why he had to have all these examinations. And I wondered if he could withstand the impact of all he had been through and emerge able to cope and be free—free to find himself, free to be the person we knew he could be.

Dr. Kenyon was visibly distressed by Tim's response. He

questioned me about the drugs Tim had previously taken. He wrote a new prescription for one of them. "I will not over-drug any child to make him livable or turn him into a classroom vegetable!" he stated firmly.

Tim came home tense every day the first few weeks of school. "I don't have any friends to play with," he complained.

"How's your teacher?" I asked.

"She's nice, Mom. She helps me."

"We could ask her to help you find a friend."

Mrs. Davis proved to be the warm and understanding person we had prayed for. She helped Tim find a friend and kept us posted about how he was doing, through mini-conferences and phone calls.

She possessed an inner patience and a firm quality to which children responded. Her creative ideas motivated Tim in positive ways. His anxiety diminished as he began to trust her and as he sensed success in his schoolwork.

In late October Mrs. Johnson, the principal, called. "I've been observing Tim in the classroom. Despite his problems, Tim works hard to succeed and wants to be like children his age. He is becoming more self-confident, less anxious, and is contributing to the class," she concluded.

"Thank you, Lord," I prayed gratefully.

A few days later, Tim bounced into the house. "Mom, guess what?" he yelled. "I've earned ten happy faces at school. All I need is ten more to get a special award."

I put my arms around him. "That's great! How about helping yourself to a special *Mom* award of homemade cookies and milk?"

Tim dumped his books on the table and pulled out his school papers. "Look, Mom, I got a 100 percent on all these papers except these two! I goofed," he said with mock seriousness. "The work is really cinchy. It's lots easier than last year. Mrs. Davis is nice to me. She helps me with my work. Not like last year," he added with a frown. "My teacher screamed at me all the time!"

"Last year is past."

"I know, but I sure wish I didn't have to take third grade over again. I flunked!"

"You didn't flunk. Your school passed you to fourth grade. Dad and I felt you should repeat third grade. We thought it would help you."

"If my teacher hadn't gotten mad at me, maybe I'd be in fourth grade," he challenged.

"Tim," I picked up his papers, "see how well you're doing this year."

As he rushed out the door to play, turbulent thoughts of the past troubled me. I had to remind myself that although the past seemed unbelievable, the present was an answer to our prayers.

On November 5, Mrs. Davis phoned. "Tim was sharing in front of the class, and in the middle of a sentence he stopped suddenly and dropped his hands to his sides. He stood staring blankly for a minute and then he was able to complete his story."

Tim hadn't arrived home yet, but in a few seconds he was in the door. He was frightened and immediately began to tell me what happened. It shocked him so much that he kept repeating, "I'll never share in front of the class again."

I tried to reassure him, "It probably will never happen again." But he remained adamant, and it was another year before he had the courage to participate in sharing time again.

I sensed that this was not just an ordinary forget-where-I-am-so-I-stop-and-think experience. Because of Tim's bewilderment and the teacher's concern, I called Dr. Kenyon, who instructed me, "Watch Tim closely. Have his teacher do likewise. Inform me if this happens again. This may have been a mild seizure, and if it occurs again another EEG will be necessary."

On Friday afternoon several weeks later Tim bounced in the door. His Raggedy-Andy hair flopped in his eyes and fringed his freckled face.

"Guess what, Mom! Only two more happy faces and I'll have twenty!"

He could hardly wait to return to school Monday morning. He was sure that by the end of the week he would earn them all.

The next Thursday afternoon the front door crashed open. Tim was home.

"Hi, Tim," I sang out. "How'd it go today?"

A thud hit the floor. "Awful! Just awful!" he cried angrily.

"What happened?"

A garble of words erupted.

"I don't understand what you're saying."

His teeth clenched; he struck the air with his fist. "I have twenty faces and I won't get my award."

"How come?"

He answered, but his words were distorted and senseless.

I put my hand on his shoulder. "Tim, let's call your teacher and find out. Maybe you didn't understand the rules."

Just then the phone rang. It was Mrs. Davis. "Tim ran out of the class. Do you know what could have happened to make him so upset?"

"He thought he would get a special award when he earned twenty faces."

"No wonder he was upset," she replied. "It takes fifty happy faces to earn it."

"What did she say, Mom?" Tim asked.

"She said that you need to earn fifty happy faces."

"I'll never earn it," he moaned. "That will take forever."

"I know you have a hard time waiting, Tim. You'll be surprised. Time will pass faster than you realize."

As the weeks went by, Tim proudly showed us his school papers. He never mentioned the award and we felt it better not to ask.

Christmas truly brought joy to our world. Tim sang with his class in the all-school Christmas program. He told his teacher that I played the Autoharp, and she invited me to come and sing Christmas music with the children. We sang the traditional carols and all their favorites. Tim was proud that I could come and be a part of his school. It gave him a sense of belonging and importance.

For a Christmas gift his grandmother made him a white doctor's coat, which he had requested. Among other toys he received a doctor's bag. He wore his white coat, used his stethoscope, shot dispenser, and candied pills to pretend he was the doctor dispensing medicine and giving shots to his patients, the two surviving teddy bears.

The last Monday in January Tim danced into the house. Jumping up and down, he exclaimed, "Close your eyes! Now put your hands out." He placed a piece of paper on my hand. "Open your eyes and see what it is."

I opened my eyes to see a small bright orange envelope with "Mr. and Mrs. Cragg" neatly inscribed on the front. Tim's eyes danced. "Open it and see what it says," he giggled. On the back was a small black "O" with two dots for eyes and a half circle smile inside. Printed next to it was, "Smile, today is your day!"

Above it, half printed and half written, were scrawled, "Smile, God loves you."

Inside was a large yellow circle with another happy face covering the whole page.

"Hurry up, read it, Mom. What does it say?"

"On the front under the smile it says, 'Keep up the good work, Tim!' " I turned it over and read the note aloud to him.

Dear Mr. and Mrs. Cragg,

I am pleased to announce that your son, Tim, has earned the "Happy Face" award. He has earned this award by collecting fifty happy face cards for good behavior and for getting his work done.

You can be proud of your son for earning this award.

Sincerely,
Mrs. Davis

We hugged each other and danced up and down, shouting and talking all at the same time. "Oh, Tim, you got your award! Your dad will be so proud."

"The teacher gave it to me just before school was over. Only *four* kids got one, and she gave it to us in front of the *whole class*!"

I turned the envelope over. "Tim, when did you write this on here?"

Taking it out of my hand, he said, "Before I left class." Pointing to each word with his finger, slowly, distinctly he read, "Smile, God loves you."

I wrapped my arms around him and pulled his feet up off the floor. "Yes, He loves you. And I'm so glad you know it!"

9

A Third EEG

The last of February Tim secretly secluded himself in the garage every day after school. After three days he came out of hiding and proudly produced a one-page typewritten letter to his friend Bob, who had come to visit. Then he also typed a one-page letter to his dad, who was setting up an auto parts warehouse in Nevada.

Writing stories or expressing himself on paper had been impossible for Tim the previous year. He had written a short camp letter, but this was the first time he'd composed two full typewritten pages. I was pleased with Tim's surprise.

Tim opened his letter by inscribing the closing salutation on top of the page.

> Love, Tim C.
>
> dear dad i miss you a hole lot. i wish you were here at home. i cant believe how long you were gone march 3 i am going to a carnival me and Kevin are getting a long good i am haveing fun with my friends i hope you are having fun there Bob came over to see me Kevin and mom are having fun i had to almost had to stay after school i think i got another girl friend i have an office of my own it is in the garage i bought a stapler i can't

hardly wait tell you get home.

In March, Tim complained that he was having headaches and seeing different colored spots and stars. At first when I talked to Dr. Kenyon I thought Tim was reacting to the drug as he had before, but intuitively I felt there were additional difficulties.

We went to see Dr. Kenyon who questioned Tim about the spots. He asked him what color they were and what other sensations he'd been having.

He turned toward me. "He may be having petit mal seizures. We'll need to schedule him for an EEG test at Memorial Hospital right away. Have my nurse call Dr. Jones's office to set the time."

Tim began crying, his slender body slumped forward. "Not another one!" I gasped with a sense of anguish.

For the first time, Dr. Kenyon's usually relaxed, jovial manner changed. Surveying both of us, he knew he would have to take command. "Now, Tim, *stop crying*. *Mother,* this test needs to be done."

"But they put needles in your brain," Tim protested.

"Not anymore. They have round discs, which they attach to your head with clay. They no longer use a machine with needles."

Tim and I felt dismayed. We were two unhappy, defenseless people. Unsteadily we left the office arm in arm. The hospital was adjacent to Dr. Kenyon's office.

"Tim, why don't we walk over to the hospital and see if we can look at the new machine?"

We went into the emergency entrance and I explained to the receptionist why we were there. She responded to our request with consideration, despite the fact that they were very busy. She called the technician, who took us to where the EEG would be administered.

The technician explained how the machine worked and showed Tim the round flat discs. I thanked her for her kindness and we left.

Ironically, for the third time, this EEG test would be taken once again in the month of April. But when we told Ron that evening, he firmly announced that he would not allow Tim to go through it again. Ron had made a promise that he intended to keep. After hearing about the new type of machine and the possibility of epilepsy, Ron recognized that the test had to be done, and reluctantly consented.

We asked Tim what type of recreation he would like to do to help him stay awake. He chose bowling. We waited until eight o'clock to look for an alley where we could bowl. We did not know that it was league night, and we searched for an hour and a half and couldn't find a bowling alley that wasn't filled to capacity. By nine-thirty we couldn't think of anything to do, until Tim finally suggested miniature golf.

The night was cold and clear. We had to keep moving to stay warm. Sometimes the boys hit their balls too far, and they'd have to retrieve them out of water traps or at another hole. The moving traps, miniature houses, whirling objects, ramps, and jumps fascinated the boys.

We tallied our scores before we played the final eighteenth hole. I have always been uncoordinated when it comes to golf and have yet to win anything more than last place. This night was no exception. Tim placed third, Kevin second, and Ron, who's always been a pro at this game, won first place.

Tim was disgusted. "This has been a cruddy day. We couldn't bowl. And I only got third place here." Disheartened, he swung at his last ball. "Brrinnng!" A red light flashed and Tim had won a free game!

Because Tim was older this time, the stay-awake marathon was not the ordeal of the past. He went to school the next day because the test was not until 2:30 P.M. By the time I picked Tim up, he was tired, troubled, and uneasy. He despised the test, and yet he knew he had to resign himself to it.

The hospital was a thirty-minute drive away. Neither Tim nor I had much to say. What was there to talk about? I detested the test for him as much as he hated it, and we both knew it.

Two weeks later I called Dr. Kenyon's office to learn the outcome of the EEG. He informed me that it was completely normal, with no abnormal brain wave patterns. He wasn't sure what caused the dizzy spells. I was pleased with the results, but on the other hand I was perplexed. Why had we needed to subject Tim to this test again? It seemed so senseless.

10

Birthday, Bicycle, and Big Bear

When Christmas is over Tim starts his birthday requests, and when his birthday passes, he begins his Christmas list. Our Sears toy catalog is always threadbare, torn, curled, and marked up from overuse.

Birthdays, Christmas, and all holidays are cherished by Tim. The pre-planning, pre-wishing, and pre-hoping are as much a part of the celebration to him as the actual day, which quite often is anticlimactic compared to his dreams for it.

One thing is certain. Tim's persistent requests and determination that this is exactly what he wants today will surely change tomorrow. On this particular year since Christmas, however, one item remained on the top of his birthday list—a new bicycle with gears to give it speed and class. He decided he had outgrown his old bike.

His grandparents usually ask Tim what he wants, and this year Tim suggested money for a bicycle. After his birthday we pooled his monetary gifts and I took him to the store to pick out a bicycle.

What an agonizing decision. It took Tim a long time to select a metallic green three-speed model. Tim was so excited when we picked up the unassembled bike from the warehouse that his hands shook. He bounced and jumped up and down in the backseat of the car, talking a mile-a-minute.

Tim watched intently while Ron sorted the bike parts. His dad showed him how to tighten the bolts and together they assembled the bicycle.

Although Tim had ridden a bike since he was five-and-a-half, he wobbled on his new one because he couldn't coordinate gear changing, gripping the brakes, and looking at the same time. He missed parked cars by a whisper or forgot to watch for oncoming cars. We were positive that if he didn't learn to look, as well as shift, he'd collide with a car.

We had always expected Tim to ride his bicycle on the streets close to home because he didn't have confidence in his own sense of direction and he was afraid of getting lost.

But one Saturday Tim thought he'd fly his independence wings on his new bicycle. I had planned to take Tim with me to pick up Kevin, who had stayed all night with a friend. I expected him to be riding nearby. When I went out to look, I couldn't find him.

"Tim, come home! Tim. Tim, come home!" I called. I was sure that if he didn't hear me, the neighbors would send him home.

I walked up and down the street looking and calling, but no Tim. I checked with his friend Anthony, questioning him at length. He finally confessed that Tim had gone to dirt hills, near a market a mile away.

I got in the car and drove down the street to where I was sure Tim would be. I circled around the store but Tim was nowhere in sight. On my way back home I drove slowly up and down the side streets, sure that I'd find Tim on one of them.

When I arrived home and Tim wasn't there, I prayed that I'd find him. This time I drove a different route to the market. Still no Tim.

I drove slowly toward home. For a second time I checked all the side streets. When I pulled into the driveway, Tim was nowhere in sight.

God's quiet voice urged me not to panic but to wait. I

decided I'd vacuum the floors. With each push forward of the cleaning wand I prayed that God would impress Tim to come home. With each stroke backward I feared that something had happened to him.

Just as I had completed my cleaning session, a thud hit the front door. It burst open. Breathlessly Tim exclaimed, "I'm scared to death! I just had to get home!"

"How come?" I asked as casually as I could manage.

His eyes widened. "Something inside of me made me feel I had to get home. I was afraid I'd get into trouble."

By now I had calmed down enough to remind Tim what his bicycle boundaries were. Then I informed him that his bike would be banished to the garage for the rest of the day and for two more days.

Tim didn't like having his wings clipped and protested the loss of his bike. At first he just complained, and then he threatened to sneak his bicycle and ride it anyhow. The rest of the afternoon I watched him closely. I sensed he was heading for an angry outburst.

Tim thought his dad would lift the restriction when he came home from work. Ron agreed with my decision and told Tim he couldn't take off like that again. Tim's already electric emotions unleashed into an intense screaming tirade.

Tim stomped into his bedroom. Ron followed, took off his belt, and spanked Tim. He had never used a belt on Tim before. We knew physical punishment had not worked in the past, but Ron felt Tim's tantrum was a get-my-own-way manipulation tactic. He thought the shock of a sound spanking would snap Tim out of it.

Ron was unnerved when he came out of the bedroom. His punishment hadn't penetrated Tim. It was as if Ron had spanked a blank, unmovable wall. Tim remained untouched; his rage continued unchecked. It took both Ron and me to prevent Tim from demolishing his room or hurting himself or us.

School came to a close in mid-June, and Tim brought home

his finest report card ever. He was proud of his progress, but was especially excited that Mrs. Davis had also been promoted to fourth grade and would be his teacher again.

In July our family planned to spend a week at Big Bear Lake. Vacations are our time of renewal. The change of scenery relaxes us all. We are not pressured by the usual demands of daily living and we can escape some of the routine stresses we all endure. Tim thrives in the out-of-doors and is totally tranquilized by a camping environment. Afterwards, he loves to talk about these oasis times and relive them.

The A-frame cabin we rented had a shiny lacquered knotty pine exterior with a front porch. It was nestled off the road, and a dry creek bed carved its way across and down beside it.

Inside, the cabin was carpeted with gold shag tweed. The brick fireplace, knickknacks, antiques, and furniture made it a lovely country home.

A friend had rented it to us for the unusually reasonable amount of fifty dollars for the week. We were grateful God had provided this haven for us.

Early the next morning we watched out the wall of windows that looked across the porch. Holes had been cut in the floor of the porch to accommodate two pine trees. Stellar jays perched on the slender branches and gray squirrels with feather duster tails scampered up and down the tree trunks.

The stellar jays' iridescent wings, black breasts, and crew-cut feathered heads danced from side to side. They darted about snatching peanuts. Then they'd perch close to the window and scold as a mother to her child. "Don't move. Stay right there." Sneaking another peanut, they'd fly away.

The squirrels joined this peanut-snitching brigade of birds. They scurried within a few inches of the door, grabbed a peanut, and scampered onto the porch railing. Protecting their territory from this invasion, the birds swooped down like dive bombers just above the squirrels' heads. The squirrels squeaked and hissed, stole the peanuts anyway, and scooted off the porch.

Kevin and Tim delighted in watching the continuous war for peanuts between the squawking jays and the squeaking squirrels.

We toured the lake, strolled through the town, and window-shopped. The boys went on a short horseback ride. A small observatory is based on a narrow peninsula that juts into the lake. We climbed up the winding stairs into the steel-encased laboratory and watched films of eruptions and explosions on the sun's surface. At twilight we rode bicycles, and in the evening we played table games.

By midweek a case of fishing fever set in. It was warm. Sunrays touched the lake like fireworks, shooting sparks of light everywhere. Waves rippled across the lake and tickled the sandy shore.

The fish were biting and the boys were exhilarated every time they caught one. A few seconds later they groaned when one got away.

By the end of our stay, they had become expert fishermen. They knew just where to cast their lines and the type of hooks and bait to use. They caught an average of fifteen fish a day, and insisted that twenty had escaped.

On Friday evening the boys wanted to fish as late as possible. They didn't want to leave, even to eat dinner, because they knew this was their last opportunity. We were leaving Saturday. I drove to the store to buy them more bait and get them a snack.

All day Tim had not budged from his perch on the rocks. Ordinarily he would have been fidgety and fussy after ten hours of just sitting, but nothing would pry him loose.

When the boys finally gave up, it was pitch dark. Only the moon cast its shadow across the face of the water. I had no idea that they had caught so many fish. At the cabin we had to fill every pot and kettle we could find.

It was late at night by the time Ron and the boys cleaned the last of the fish. We stuffed as many as we could in the freezer. We had fish, fish, and more fish. We would have to bake them, fry them, freeze them, and give them away.

While we drove down the mountain the boys chattered, reliving the vivid details of how the fish managed to wiggle off their hooks. They talked about the ones they saw jumping out of the lake, or those they snagged but didn't catch. The happy memories of that week would linger with them for a long time.

11

A Sunshine Summer and Simba

The remainder of the summer a conglomeration of neighborhood children converged on our yard. The gang played assorted games like football and basketball, and at night they played flashlight tag, ding-dong ditchum, and snake in the grass.

In late July they decided to plan a carnival. It took three full days to set it up because the gang tried out all the games to make sure they worked. There were cans to knock down, basketballs to throw into barrels, bowling pins to belt, and a fortune wheel. Sponges sopped in shaving cream were the weapons used to throw at whoever would volunteer to stick his face out of a hole in a big painted box. Along the back of the house they set up a game prize and refreshment booth.

Thursday morning the motley menagerie gathered in their costumes. Wearing a black top hat, our neighbor boy, John, led the parade on his bicycle. He was the barker and his ear-piercing voice bellowed through his paper bullhorn.

"Come to the carnival! Come to the carnival!"

"Boom! Boom! Boom!" Tim's drum echoed.

The straggling band of offbeat marchers paraded down the

street beckoning all to join them. Come they did! In droves! In herds! In flocks! Tall and small, child and adult descended upon us.

When the crowd thinned out, the workers played the games themselves. They tromped in and out of the house to replenish their food supply. Trails of popcorn and lemonade trickled across the floor. Our tiny two-bedroom house and yard were decorated in early-American bedlam.

I hibernated inside and watched the beehive of activity buzzing outside. Tim couldn't handle the confusion. He flitted from game to game instead of staying where he belonged. Every so often he'd come in to tattle. Tim expected me to straighten out whoever he thought was not doing things the way he thought they should. When I couldn't agree with him, he'd stomp out and take things into his own hands, and a squabble was sure to start.

The chaos of the carnival was too much. By the time it closed, Tim spiraled into a state of agitated explosiveness. When our quiet returned, Tim calmed down.

Throughout the summer Tim had been talking about wanting a puppy. He fantasized stories about having a German shepherd. "I can teach the dog to pin and kill robbers," he'd declare, imagining would-be break-ins. But we weren't sure we were ready for a dog.

Ron finally relented, with a few stipulations, "Tim, you'll have to earn enough money to buy the puppy and to pay for all the necessary shots."

Tim agreed immediately, "I will! I will!"

"And you'll have to be responsible for feeding, cleaning up after, and taking care of the dog. The puppy has to be a male, stay outside, and be medium size or small when it grows up." Ron measured the size in the air with his hands to emphasize what size medium was. "And it's not to be a German shepherd." Ron punctuated each word to accent his final point.

Tim jumped up and down. "How can I earn the money?"

"Well, you can start by trimming the hedge. Then we can think of some chores," I suggested.

Tim dashed to the garage, got out the clippers, then came back to the living room. "Mom, mark the hedge off with a rag so I can have something to work for."

I tied a blue rag to a section about five feet from where Tim planned to begin. With long-handled clippers, a saw, and short nippers, Tim clipped, snipped and sawed away at our 120-foot hedge. Diligently he persevered. When he reached the marker, he'd whoop into the house, waving the rag triumphantly like a flag.

With the goal of reaching the rag spurring him on, he'd work for two or three hours at a time. In two days the hedge was trimmed and he asked, "What else can I do now?"

"You could trim the red berry bush," I volunteered.

Outside our back door stood a six-foot high by three-foot square berry bush. During the summer it was decorated with lacy white flowers and its red berries set it aflame at Christmas. Knowing that Tim was in an exuberant mood I should have maintained a closer eye on his trimming. Employed in household chores, however, I ignored what he was doing.

After completing his clipping session, he raced in and exclaimed, "Come see my work. I'm finished!"

He made me close my eyes as he led me out to see his handiwork. To my surprise, nothing was left of our bush except the huge stump. Beaming triumphantly, he announced, "See what I did!"

He was so proud, I didn't have the heart to tell him he'd overdone it a bit.

It was the weekend so we put the dog-seeking adventure off until Monday. August 13 was one of those golden tinsel-and-glitter sunshine days for which California is famous. The sun's blinding brightness gave the pavement a slick-as-cellophane appearance. Rays reflecting against glass and steel winked at us. Our car sped along the concrete freeways which slither in, out, and all over California like slender snakes. We took the off-ramp that ended at the combination dog pound, county facilities, and men's jail.

At the guard station a trustee directed us toward the long rows of chain-link fenced cages. As we wandered down the central mall, dogs on both sides of us barked, danced, and jumped at us. Their yowls, yipes, barks, and growls sounded like an off-key musical production which they were directing offbeat with their wagging tails.

We wandered through the long row of cages twice, but none of the puppies seemed to spark that special feeling that says, "That's the one."

Tim was overanxious and disconcerted that he couldn't find a puppy. He began to cry and wanted to choose just any dog. The Humane Society was another forty minutes from where we were, and I finally convinced him to at least go there and look.

When we arrived at the Humane Society I told Tim that I wanted him to explain what he wanted. When Tim tries to express his wants or wishes to someone else, he finds it almost impossible. He relies on others to communicate his desires. Lately I'd encouraged Tim to state his own requests. Although it was painful to watch him fumble and falter for words, I knew it was essential.

Kevin and I stood behind Tim as he asked the officer, "Do you have any puppies we can buy? How much do they cost?"

The officer pointed toward a door and told him, "A small pen of puppies is located in the center yard."

It was an instant love affair between Tim and a brown puppy. The pup jumped, yipped, wiggled all over, and had that "pick me up" appeal in his eyes. His ears were pointed and his long slender nose and mouth were black. He was rusty brown, with white paws and breast, and the tip of his long tail was fringed in grease-spot black.

He looked like he was a German shepherd mix. I knew we should find out before we decided that he was the one we wanted.

The officer said, "Yes, the dog is part shepherd, and I don't know what else."

"How big do you think he will get?" I questioned.

The officer measured the size he thought the dog would grow with his hand held above the desk top. It looked about the size Ron had measured in the air at home.

"Can we return him if he's not okay with our dad?" the boys inquired.

The officer assured us, "Up to thirty days you can return the pup in exchange for another one."

An inner judgment battle raged. *Should I or shouldn't I take the pup home when he is part German shepherd? Tim will be unbearably upset if we have to bring the dog back.*

As we stood and looked at the puppies again, I'm afraid that the pup's brown eyes and appealing personality, coupled with two excited boys, overruled.

The pup knew to whom he belonged at once, and rested his head on Tim's lap. Dogs, cats, and most animals form an instant bond with Tim because their instincts can sense the unspoken "spirit of love" that Tim generates.

All the way home we discussed a name for our new dog. Somewhere between the Humane Society and home we settled on "Simba."

The rest of the day Tim played with, cradled, and showed off Simba to his friends until the poor pup became so sick that I had to tell Tim, "You'll have to find something else to do. Puppies, like babies, need naps." Exhausted, Simba slept soundly for a long time.

At 5:30 P.M. Ron drove in the driveway; the fateful hour had arrived when Father would see the new puppy. Tim raced out to the car with Simba. Within a matter of seconds the pup won Ron over, and Simba was here to stay.

Ron let us know however, "You were duped by the Humane Society officer. Look at the puppy's paws." Ron picked up the puppy's paw to point out its size. "The dog will be much bigger than you were told, and the German shepherd part has almost completely taken over whatever mix the dog was supposed to have."

I claimed honest innocence. "I didn't know that paw size is an indicator of dog size. But I must admit that Simba's paws are pretty big for a six-week-old puppy. The officer said we could exchange him for another one."

"No, no, we'll keep the dog," Ron muttered, picked up the evening paper, and began to shuffle through it. I'm sure Ron didn't want to suffer through broken hearts any more than I did.

Since Simba was to stay outside, and puppies usually cry at night, Tim asked if he and our neighbor boy, John, could sleep out in our two-man backpacker's tent to keep the dog company.

The exuberant puppy pulled on the strings, uprooted the stakes, and then sat on the tent. At first Tim and John laughed at silly Simba. They pushed the dog out of the way, put the stakes back into the ground, and straightened the tent.

Before they could crawl into their sleeping bags for the night, the untrained puppy soiled John's bag. Both boys scolded Simba, and John had to go home to get something else to sleep in.

The puppy stimulated Tim, and he began to wind up out of control. We had to calm Tim down and remind him that Simba was only a puppy.

I finally suggested that the boys tie Simba up just short of the tent where he could be next to it but not on top of it or in it.

The next night Tim wanted to sleep outside again, but we knew that Simba should learn to sleep alone. No sooner had our family settled down for the night when the whimpering cry of a motherless pup penetrated our bedroom.

"He'll quit in a few minutes," we told ourselves.

A few minutes stretched into thirty. We lay awake, hoping Simba would stop. Tim kept pleading, "Can't I sleep outside? Simba's lonely. Can't he come in?"

Our puppy's lusty voice wailed louder and louder. Beside me, Ron lay stiffly, mumbling. "This is why I didn't want a dog. I have to work tomorrow. If the blasted dog doesn't stop, our friendly neighbors won't be so friendly."

And so our outside dog became an inside dog. We corraled Simba in the boys' room and put a box of dirt on the rug, hoping the pup would properly use it. Instead, Simba sniffed the box, pounced into it, and with both paws dug vigorously, spraying dirt all over the carpet. The boys giggled. Ron grumbled. We removed the box, vacuumed, and put down newspapers. Exhausted by the excitement, Simba curled up next to Tim's bed and quickly fell asleep.

We woke in the morning to find that the pup had christened the carpet, chewed on the newspapers, and strewn them everywhere. The next few weeks our nightly calisthenics consisted of laying a complete coverage of newspapers over the carpet, along with a thorough toy-and-clothes cleanup campaign.

The boys learned the hard way that any treasure that could be destroyed by a puppy's teeth would have to be stored out of reach. Simba especially loved socks and furry stuffed toys. More than once we'd waken to find a toy in bite-size pieces or socks with holes chewed in them.

It was several weeks before our new baby was housebroken. There was a lot of growling around our house, but not from the dog. Ron didn't think he'd survive Simba's infancy.

12

Drowned in a Turbulent Sea of Changes

Stimulating changes had been taking place in our lives, and the effects were fraying at the edge of Tim. He was spiraling completely out of control.

Our country-type church had never grown, secluded in its back-street area. We had hired a new pastor the previous year to assist us in selling and relocating our church.

Our church property finally sold, and by midsummer we had moved out and rented a civic-center facility. Another struggling congregation merged with us because they were selling their poorly located property also.

Our once small congregation had now doubled in size. Tim felt lost and out of place in the new surroundings, with new people. Tim was unable to play freely. His hideouts were gone. Trees to climb and a place to let off steam harmlessly no longer existed.

Tim rebelled on Sunday mornings while we were getting ready for church. He stormed belligerently and begged, "Let me stay home! I don't want to go. I hate church! It's boring!"

While driving to church he became even more upset because we gave a ride to Johnny Orr, a forty-year-old man from our former church. Johnny had a speech impediment, limped, and had never been able to go to school. When our church relocated, he could no longer walk, and we promised him a ride to our new facility. Johnny's deep faith and love for the Lord enriched our lives.

Tim couldn't cope with Johnny's deformities. He had always mimicked Johnny's speech and walk. "Ahh—dahh. Johnny Orr, Johnny Orr, Johnny Orr," Tim parroted and slurred his words, then limped and lurched in Johnny's unsteady gait.

Tim became increasingly disturbed by Johnny's presence in our car. I spent most of our ride to church silently preventing Tim from mimicking Johnny. Both Ron and I tried to help Tim understand, be compassionate, and realize his make-fun behavior was cruel. But the more Johnny rode with us, the worse Tim became. After repeatedly attempting to stop Tim, we had to make other transportation arrangements for Johnny.

A square-shaped pond and waterfall which adjoined the civic-center building was the kind of bait that attracted boys. We tried to watch Tim to keep him off the fountain and from throwing rocks into it.

Tim's behavior was impulsive. He never thought of the consequences of this behavior. Someone was always reprimanding him or reminding him to stay out of the fountain and to respect the buildings.

Tim picked fights and threw rocks at boys he'd never met from the other congregation. We were forever breaking up Tim's fights or being summoned to stop one.

The only church activity to which Tim seemed somewhat able to adjust was the junior Sunday School class taught by Walt Taylor. Tim was distracted and often disruptive. But Walt's patience and persistence at trying to find ways to reach Tim finally began to conquer. Walt took David and Tim out to dinner, and together they devised ways that Sunday School could be made more appealing. Walt had chosen the evening-out idea to capture Tim's interest and motivate him toward self-control in class.

Tim's hostile attitude and silent refusal to participate in another class for his age group upset the program to such a degree that we finally had to stop taking him. We felt helpless. I'm sure that people who didn't know us or Tim thought he was an undisciplined brat.

Another gradual change had been happening on our home front. Unexpected waves of infection and pain plagued and fatigued me. My only recourse was rest in bed until they subsided. Although I was under the care of two specialists and taking pain medication and antibiotics, the exact cause of my continued bladder infections had not been determined.

Shortly after school started in September I stopped by to see Mrs. Davis. She seemed puzzled. "I've noticed a marked difference in Tim from last year. He's uncooperative and unable to do skills or work he could handle in third grade. His favorite friends have moved away, and instead of trying to make new ones he's become withdrawn."

At home Tim complained that he had headaches, was dizzy, and his eyes crossed unexpectedly. He was touchy, moody, and lethargic. His temper flared and he wept, whined, and wailed at the least provocation.

Super-active Simba continued to disrupt our household, and we began to wonder if we could keep him. Although his antics were cute, they agitated all of us.

When Tim and Kevin dressed for school, the pup would grab one of the boys' socks just as he was about to put it on. Then Simba would jump on the couch, hold the sock under his paw, roll his big brown eyes, wag his tail, and wait for the boys to come after the sock. Simba would steal any object he knew was important, and off he'd run in his game of hide-and-seek.

One morning Simba snatched Tim's beige teddy bear and chewed holes in it. Tim became so angry that he pummeled the puppy with his fists. No amount of scolding seemed to get through to Simba, and our inside dog had to be kept outside.

We were not sure whether Tim was overwhelmed by the stimulating summer, his new dog, the church change, the vacation-to-school transition, a reaction to the drug he was taking, or my illness. To the rest of us this tide of ebb-and-flow circumstances had gradually submerged us in a sea of our own adjustments. What we did not know was that Tim was drowning in the turbulent tidal wave of changes that flooded our lives. We were unable to rescue Tim or help him reach a stable shore.

On September 25, we went to see Dr. Kenyon. Tim was restless. He rocked back and forth, rubbing his hands up and down his legs. Tim told Dr. Kenyon he was upset with school because he didn't have any friends. The doctor had a long talk with Tim on how to go about making friends.

After Tim went to the waiting room, we talked at length about the changes in Tim. Dr. Kenyon told me, "I don't feel Tim is having a reaction to the drug. Tim has gained a lot of weight and has grown taller, so the drug is no longer effective. I'll fill out a prescription for the same drug, but I'll double the dosage."

(At this time we didn't know that Tim was actually taking the wrong drug or that the added dosage would continue to increase his sometimes odd behavior and intensify his hyperactivity.)

Dr. Kenyon sighed; what he had to say was not easy. "These changes in Tim can no longer be handled medically. His problems are beyond my scope. I feel you should pursue psychological counseling for Tim."

A total sense of hopelessness encompassed me. How could we afford psychological services? Our budget was stretched beyond its limit because of other medical bills and the rise in living costs. We had no extras in our monthly income. I was too ill to work. The gynecologist was still trying to correct the physical problems I was having, the urologist was medicating me for bladder infections, and a possible major surgery was pending in the future. Ron's sales schedule was erratic because he was sometimes sent to other states to work for a week or two, and he couldn't take on extra employment.

The preschool where I had previously worked had a professional consultant service. For twenty-eight dollars we could obtain four visits with a psychologist, but beyond that, the prospects were dim for continued care.

Dr. Walters had been recommended to me by the parents of several children I'd had in preschool. I'd been told that Dr. Walters had given them a complete written report about their children plus practical specific guidance, which was something we had never had before.

In the past the professionals had peered over their test results, only giving us bits and snatches of information, avoiding labels or direct statements. It was as if they'd been sworn to some secret cult.

On the afternoon of October 2 I had an appointment to consult with Dr. Walters. When faced with this type of meeting, something inside makes me clam up and block out what I want to express. I knew the only way I would remember everything was to write it out. I thought through what I wanted to say, Ron and I talked it over, and then I typed a thorough two-page report. We needed answers, and I hoped that we could get an honest evaluation and new direction without the cat-and-mouse games of the past.

Dr. Walters' waiting room was filled with mothers who chattered openly. A small door in the wall was open, and inside was a cupboard full of toys which spilled over the floor. The brothers and sisters of children who were in therapy played freely with chalkboards, building blocks, and other toys on the rug. It was a warm, relaxed place to be, and I rested a little easier.

Dr. Walters was an easygoing, quiet, slow-speaking man who thought carefully while talking. He was dressed in slacks, colored shirt, tie, and casual suede shoes, which were popular with the youth. He set me at ease immediately.

I handed Dr. Walters the typewritten report and waited while he read it. When he had finished reading, he asked me questions about Tim's EEG tests.

After a lengthy discussion about Tim's medical and behavioral history, Dr. Walters summarized our conversation. "It would be my belief that Tim has what is called a subclinical convulsive syndrome. I've been working for a long time with children with this form of epilepsy. Even though Tim's last two brain wave tests were normal, the fact that the first EEG showed epileptic patterns, coupled with what you've told me about his behavior, strongly indicates that Tim has this nonconvulsive form of epilepsy."

As our conversation came to a close, we agreed that I would bring Kevin and Tim in next. Then Dr. Walters would see Tim alone, and finally he would consult with Ron and me. Dr. Walters gave me a list of books to read, but especially urged me to read Dr. Walter C. Alvarez's book *Nerves in Collision*.

Kevin was unsure about visiting a psychologist. "How come I have to see a shrink?" he questioned sarcastically. His jabbing remark was only a cover-up for his fears. All these years Kevin had stood in the shadow of Tim's experience and he wanted no part of it. Secretly, he feared something would be the matter with him. It took a lot of explaining to help Kevin understand that the only way we could help Tim was for all of us to see Dr. Walters.

Tim was even more bewildered. He didn't perceive that a psychologist was not a physician, and kept pleading, "I don't want to go. Please don't make me go. They'll give me a shot and make me have another brain wave test."

I tried to assure Tim by reminding him of his past experience with the psychologists who only gave him learning tests, but he still opposed going. In Tim's mind all doctors were mixed together, and he didn't really care what kind they were. He didn't want to see any of them. His final pronouncement was, "I'm not going!"

On the afternoon of October 8 I took two reluctant, restless boys with me to see Dr. Walters. Kevin was sensitive, quiet, and nervous, despite his attempt to act self-assured. Tim was high-strung. He bounced and moved around the waiting room aimlessly.

I introduced the boys to Dr. Walters, who then motioned to Kevin, "You can come in first."

"Can I go outside to ride the elevator?" Tim asked me.

"No, you stay here. There are some toys over there in that cupboard." I pointed to the closed door in the wall. I knew Tim would run off if I let him outside.

Tim fumbled through the toys and thumbed through some books, but nothing pleased him. Trying to contain Tim prior to a doctor's visit is an ordeal, and it relieved me when Kevin came out and Tim was called in.

A grin of relief spread across Kevin's face, and he relaxed now that the interview was over. "Dr. Walters is nice," he admitted. "I like him. That wasn't as bad as I thought it would be."

On October 15 I took Tim in for extensive testing. The following Friday, Ron and I went to see Dr. Walters. Ron was able to talk openly and objectively with the doctor. For most of the session we discussed our home life, our personalities, and our feelings.

Dr. Walters concluded, "I believe Tim has a subclinical convulsive syndrome and should be put on a drug for epilepsy instead of the one he is now taking. I'll contact Dr. Kenyon. Tim should be brought in for individual therapy, followed by group therapy, for an indefinite time."

In the past Dr. Baldwin had indicated the possibility of epilepsy and Dr. Kenyon had suspected it. This was the first time it had been clearly defined.

Our immediate simultaneous reaction was, *How will we pay for therapy?* We simply could not afford it. Dr. Walters questioned us about our medical insurance, then told us that some health plans paid for therapy. He graciously agreed to accept whatever our insurance paid, and the rest he would write off. We knew Tim needed therapy. We knew we needed help. In faith that the bill would be paid, we agreed to go ahead.

Dr. Walters told us, "Bill, a psychiatric technician, will work with Tim from now on. I'll have follow-up consultations as they are needed."

On Monday, October 22, Dr. Walters introduced Tim and me to Bill. He was a tall and slender man with a blond complexion, sandy brown hair, and a mustache. He was wearing short boots, a light blue Levi-type shirt, and matching pants. He had an outdoorsman look, and I felt that Bill and Tim would hit it off well.

First Bill and I discussed what specific concerns I had for Tim. Lately Tim had been badgering me after school. "I have nothing to do. What's there to do?" he continuously complained. Because I was so ill, I needed Tim to motivate himself and plan his own after-school activities, despite the fact that there were other more critical areas that we needed to work on with Tim.

Tim and Bill spent twenty minutes together. When they came out, Bill explained, "I've made a contract with Tim." He handed me papers that Tim and he had filled out. "If Tim plans a half hour of his time every day, he can earn points for an award. If it's okay with Ron, Tim would like to go backpacking at O'Neil Park."

The following day when Tim came home from school, a line creased his mouth and his eyes were glazed. "Take me to the park!" he demanded.

I was completely taken off guard by his command. "But, Tim, you were supposed to plan to do something at home."

"TAKE me to the park!"

Still shocked at his emphatic statement, I repeated, "That was not in the agreement. You were to plan your day at home and then go to the park next Sunday."

"What can I do?" he blurted.

"How about mowing the lawn?"

"No—I don't want to. I don't care if I go to the park," he

sneered sarcastically.

"Why don't you get out your giant Tinker Toys?"

"No—they're toady." Tim strode over to the desk, grabbed the contract, and tore it into small pieces.

"Tim, you've destroyed your contract. That means you cannot go to the park Sunday."

"I don't care. That was a dumb plan. That stupid Bill can go jump in the lake," Tim cursed.

During the remainder of the week Tim steadily regressed. He didn't mention the contract again until Sunday morning. He came into our room extra early, plopped down on our bed, and announced, "We're going to the park to go backpacking today."

"No, we're not!" was my instant reply. "You tore up your contract. Dad and I made other plans. We're all going to visit some friends this afternoon."

Tim abruptly stood up. "I did what my contract said this week."

"Tim, you tore it up. We are *not* going to the park," Ron stated flatly.

Tim charged into his bedroom and climbed back into bed. "I'm not going to church! I'm staying home!"

Ron showered and shaved. Kevin and I dressed, and then I prepared breakfast. "Come and eat," I called from the kitchen.

"I'm not going to eat!" Tim snapped back.

Ron went into Tim's room, took him by the arm, helped him out of bed, and told him to get dressed. Ron tried to joke with Tim, hoping he could get him to laugh and bring him out of his rebellious mood. Tim continued to complain.

When I again asked Tim to come and eat, he retorted, "I'm not going to eat those dumb eggs!"

While the family ate, Tim finally finished dressing. He cursed and fussed during the entire procedure. Half the time he incoherently expressed thoughts that were disjointed and unrelated.

We finished eating and began loading the car with Sunday

School paraphernalia. Tim finished putting on his last shoe. He rose from the floor, cursed, and struck out at Ron who playfully batted back. Ron hoped that a light tussling would work out Tim's growing rampage.

Tim's agitation reached its peak at this point. SMACK! He slapped his dad soundly across the face. Ron had maintained his calm throughout this frustrating barrage of verbal abuse. But this was too much. Instantly he smacked Tim in return. "I've had enough! Stop this right now! We'll have no more!"

Tim turned and charged out the open door. He screamed, "I'm running away!" and bolted down the street.

Ron was recovering from a recent bout with the flu, and we were both washed out by the emotional stress of the morning. Neither of us moved to chase Tim. Kevin, who had quietly tried to remain unobtrusive, was deeply concerned by now. He went out in the yard to see where Tim was. Kevin shouted reports while we continued to try to gather our thoughts and take the last of our Sunday School materials to the car.

I knew Tim wouldn't stray very far away, and so I called to Kevin, "Come help me pack a lunch for Tim. He'll be hungry."

Ron went out to retrieve Tim and finally got him into the car. Tim was disheveled, his hair a stringy crumpled mass.

Ron's energy was completely sapped. Neither of us had much to say. Silently we wondered how we'd ever get through the morning.

After a while I quietly remarked, "Tim, I made you a lunch."

"No—I'm not going to eat!" he snapped.

I handed him the hairbrush. "Please brush your hair."

"No!" He put the brush down, slowly opened his sack, and eyed me to see if I was watching. He slipped his sandwich out of the plastic wrapper and devoured it. Then Tim opened his bag of corn chips, crammed a fistful at a time into his mouth, and polished off his apple and cookies.

We stopped to pick up Rod and Eric. When they got in the car, Tim laughed and talked to them as if nothing had happened. We pulled up to the church parking lot. Tim's parting shot was, "Please don't tell anyone what happened today." He jumped out of the car and bounced up the stairs to Sunday School.

Ron and I glanced at each other, sighed simultaneously, shook our heads, and got out of the car.

13

A Time of Therapy

Monday, October 29, Tim got out of school at 12:45 P.M. As we sat down to eat lunch, he announced, "I want to go to the park next Sunday. I'll plan my day and keep my contract."

"You have a session with Bill this afternoon at 3:30. You can talk to him about it then."

"I don't want to go!" he shot back.

"Tim, you can tell Bill anything you want, and how you felt about this week."

Tim mumbled, finished his lunch, and then went outside. First he pulled weeds in the flower bed and then mowed the lawn.

In the afternoon we arrived at the office. Bill popped his head through the receptionist's window. "How'd you do on your contract, Tim?"

Tim grabbed my arm, "You tell him, Mom."

"No, you have to tell Bill," I responded.

"Did you keep your contract?" Bill questioned again.

"You tell him, Mom," Tim giggled.

"Tim, you have to tell him yourself."

"I tore it up," Tim blurted.

Bill motioned through the window with his hand, "Come on. Let's go talk."

While Bill and Tim were talking, I settled down to read. The dimly lit waiting room was empty. It seemed strange and lonely without the usual echoing voices of children and adults.

Dr. Walters must have sensed the silence, because he stepped out of his office into the waiting room and glanced around. "Well, how's it going?" he queried.

"Not too well," I answered thoughtfully. "I've been wondering, Dr. Walters. What causes Tim to have the tantrums and obstinate behavior?"

"The hypothesis—and my own feeling—is that when spiking is going on—well the example that I use . . . " He spoke carefully, thinking through his words one by one. "You know on a dry day when you slide your feet across a carpet, someone touches you and it gives you a spark. How would you feel after awhile if someone did that every second to you? Psst—psst—psst, every second. You would become angry if your brain was discharging sparks and misfiring all the time. That kind of energy builds up. It's not firing off overt epileptic seizure patterns, but it fires off through anger, irritability, crankiness, temper, rage, and destructiveness."

I pondered what Dr. Walters had said and then sighed, "Yes. That makes sense to me, but there's something else that doesn't make sense. Tim fights coming to therapy, and yet he likes Bill."

Dr. Walters settled down on a footstool. "It's the inborn oppositional aspect of the syndrome."

"That's been our biggest problem all the way through," I interjected. "He opposes everything we do or want him to do."

"Well, the words are *oppositional* and *controlling*. They tend to be born that way."

"Tim was that way from birth."

"Even the nurses in the hospital will say that some little kids are born oppositional. You should read Dr. Alvarez's book *Nerves in Collision*," Dr. Walters suggested. "Get ahold of it."

"I have. I've read the whole thing. It was like reading a family history. In fact, I think my cousin and grandfather had it. I wouldn't be surprised at all—"

"You see page after page of statistics," Dr. Walters said.

"I don't remember my grandfather, but almost to the day my father died, he talked about his father's rages. And then on Ron's side of the family, his great-grandfather and five of his children had epilepsy. It's been ironic. I couldn't believe the hereditary links when I read the book."

Dr. Walters nodded. "Medical people and educators need to recognize the subclinical syndrome early. Almost all the kids' symptoms have ballooned because they have gone unrecognized. Maybe your son should have been on Dilantin from the day he was born."

"Yes. He was on epilepsy medicine for a while, and he did very well, but we never clearly understood that he had epilepsy. Now that he's on a different drug, he's regressed. Have you talked to Dr. Kenyon about changing Tim's medication to Dilantin?"

"We haven't been able to get together on the phone," he replied. "When I call Dr. Kenyon he isn't there and vice versa. I'll make sure I reach him right away," Dr. Walters assured me.

"Do they outgrow it?" I asked.

"Often they do, but sometimes it goes over into adulthood. Temporal lobe seizure patterns are pretty well established—sometimes. One boy I know was expelled from school by the school board at the age of seven because of his disruptive actions. With help, he is now at the local university doing outstanding work and is an excellent citizen."

Dr. Walters slowly rose to his feet and started toward his office. "You need to develop a good case of patience to live with these children."

When Tim came bounding out of his session with Bill, he was grinning. Bill put his arm on Tim's shoulder while they stood in front of me.

"What is our agreement?" Bill asked.

"I don't remember," Tim said.

Bill prompted Tim, but Tim still looked blank. Finally Bill repeated almost the entire sentence. "I will try not to arg—"

"Argue with my parents!" Tim blurted.

"What about last week's contract?" I questioned. "Tim still wants to earn his way to the park."

Bill turned to Tim. "That is a lot, Tim. Do you think you can do it?"

Tim nodded.

"Could I speak to you for a few minutes?" I asked Bill. Tim darted out the door; he'd been cooped up long enough. "Tim has become more rebellious since starting therapy. He opposes coming and fights everything new we try."

"Sometimes this happens because therapy is a threatening experience," Bill assured me. "Would you be willing to keep a daily diary? Maybe this would give us some insight and we could pinpoint a few things."

"Sure," I agreed. "That's an excellent idea."

"Try to write down exactly what Tim does, how he reacts, and what the family says and does in response. Keep the diary for two weeks and then we can sec what we discover from it."

By the time I reached the car, the intensity of Tim's feelings had reached a high pitch. "Hrrr-umpy—umpy—umpy," he hissed between clenched teeth. Tim attacked the car viciously, bouncing his body back and forth against the rear seat.

He threw himself against the seat in a rocking, rhythmic motion with such force that he shook the entire car. I tried to talk to Tim and divert his attention to look at the freeway jammed with work traffic or any other point of interest, but he continued.

Suddenly he crawled over the seat and sat up front. He switched on the radio, moved the dial around, then snapped his fingers and bounced his feet up and down while he listened to rock and roll music. I was so distracted by Tim that it was a wonder we arrived home safely.

The next day was Halloween. For Tim the anticipation was

unbearable. Tim didn't have to get up for school until 8:00, but he was awake and ready for Halloween at 6:00 A.M. Through that groggy fog we call sleep, we could hear the strains of "song-song blue—weeping like a willow," sung in Tim's cheerful voice. He interrupted his singing only to wake Kevin up. "Kevin. Kevin. Wake up. We have to call Rod and Eric to come over. I'm going to trick-or-treat at five o'clock tonight."

Kevin didn't respond to Tim's barrage of Halloween happiness, but gave him the brilliant idea that he should come into our room. Jumping and swaying from side to side, Tim told us, "I'm going to trick-or-treat at five o'clock."

Ron and I both mumbled, "It's too early! Go back to bed." Instead Tim left our bedroom and let Simba in the house. The dog charged for our room and scrambled onto our bed.

Ron shoved Simba off the bed. "Tim, take the dog out," he ordered. Tim took Simba to the living room. In a few minutes the dog yelped, scurried into our room, and hid under the bed.

"Tim, you're being too rough with the dog," I scolded.

Tim danced around. "I'm excited about trick-or-treating."

That's a pure understatement, if I ever heard one, I thought to myself.

By breakfast time I had become short-tempered and snapped at Tim.

"I'm going to tell Bill on you," Tim threatened. "You're not supposed to treat me this way."

Halloween Day I felt open, exposed, and irritable. I was shattered emotionally by the long, long journey we had trod. I somehow realized that tangled and intertwined in all of this were not only Tim's inborn problems, but our reactions to him.

We seemed to be riding on a Ferris wheel with a different problem sitting on each chair. My personality, the attitudes of his father, his brother, the doctors, church, school, the tests, his own inner anxieties, all spun round and round and round and we were unable to get off that moving circle and reconstruct our lives.

Every time I mentioned doctor or pills, Tim cringed. "You

say you love me. But you keep taking me to doctors and giving me pills."

His eyes were bewildered, his face creased with anxiety. Had we cared too much? Were we destroying Tim? Were we overly obsessed with his problems? I wondered if that were possible.

Ron and I discussed our traits, what we were like as children, and what we had carried into our adulthood because of some of our negative childhood experiences. We could see images of ourselves in Tim, and yet these images many times were distorted.

At times Tim's irritability, obstinacy, his teasing sense of humor, his overactivity, temperamental nature—even his I-fooled-you stories and pranks—could be considered phases that an average boy might experience. It was the extreme intensity to which he carried everything—his inability to put on the brakes and stop himself that concerned us.

Sometimes we reacted too quickly, expecting the worst from Tim. Other times we were too lenient or didn't act soon enough to prevent Tim from spiraling.

Kevin had been upset by all the changes, but only to a slight degree. He seemed to adapt. He had self-direction and became actively involved in after-school sports and boys club. He saw the church change as an adventurous challenge. Kevin seemed to understand. He didn't slide so far off-balance, or become emotionally disturbed. He could carry on, laugh things off, and adjust to the ups and downs of life.

I realized that therapy would give Tim the opportunity to expose us as he saw us. I knew changes would have to come from us—our reactions, attitudes, and the way we responded to Tim. Problems in our own personalities that we didn't know existed would have to be scrutinized. It would not be easy to see ourselves revealed, to have our lives shaken by the unknown and unexpected experiences therapy would bring.

In the early afternoon I called Dr. Kenyon, who chose to communicate with me through his secretary. "Dr. Kenyon has turned everything over to the psychologist and there is nothing he can do," she said.

Anxiously I told her, "We're desperate. We've had enough. The double dosage of medication affects Tim like a tight lid on a pot of boiling water, and the steam is seeping out of the edges. The drug subdues him and makes him groggy, but he's even more temperamental."

I continued to explain the previous day's events and that Dr. Walters had talked to Dr. Kenyon about putting Tim on an epileptic medication. We had expected to hear from him. The secretary promised me she would call me back if the doctor had any more to say.

At 3:10, Tim came in the door dragging his feet. His jacket trailed the floor behind him. His eyes were droopy, and he was grouchy. He ate a snack, then plopped himself on the couch and promptly fell asleep. He slept for over an hour.

I kept the phone lines clear hoping Dr. Kenyon would call, but the call never came. The next morning discouragement, depression, and despair took me to the depths of self-pity. I didn't want to face anyone or anything anymore.

My own physical pain came and went with increasing intensity. It was like a fire lighting my already highly flammable emotions. I wondered how we'd survive times of acute pain, of being washed out, pale, and edgy. How can you help heal a child when you need to be healed yourself?

I tried to keep how I felt from Ron. I didn't like to worry him. The pressure of Tim, and Ron's work was enough. This morning, however, he took one look at me and said, "You're sick again, aren't you?"

"How'd you know?" I asked.

"I can tell by your eyes," he replied softly. My usually deep blue eyes were a pale glassy gray, he told me, and my rosy complexion was ash white.

When Ron left for work I halfheartedly sat down to read my Bible, something I had disciplined myself to do no matter how I felt. My daily devotions fortified me.

These times of quiet meditation and prayer gave me the strength to face the day. When everything the day before had gone wrong, or a morning before-school hour was particularly jangled, or the physical pain was intense and fraying my emotions, I could hardly wait for a time of quiet. During these times of spiritual fortification, I tried to remember to pray for the needs of others, wisdom, insights to my family needs, and to think of the things I could be thankful for.

The Scripture reading in my devotional book referred me to Psalm 116. David was describing how God had saved him in sorrow.

> I love the Lord, because he hath heard my voice and my supplications. Because he hath inclined his ear unto me, therefore will I call upon him as long as I live. The sorrows of death compassed me, and the pains of hell gat hold upon me: I found trouble and sorrow.

The words filled me with hope. Tears welled within, and I prayed sincerely as I read, making the words my own prayer.

> Gracious is the Lord, and righteous; yea, our God is merciful. The Lord preserveth the simple: I was brought low, and he helped me. Return unto thy rest, O my soul . . . . I believed, therefore have I spoken: I was greatly afflicted . . . . I will offer to thee the sacrifice of thanksgiving, and will call upon the name of the Lord (Ps. 116).

Then I opened Oswald Chamber's book *My Utmost for His Highest*. It had ministered to me many times before.

> The first thing God does with us is to get us based on rugged Reality until we do not care what becomes of us individually as long as He gets His way for the purpose of His Redemption. Why shouldn't we go through heartbreaks? Through those doorways God is opening up ways of fellowship with His Son. Most of us fall and collapse at the first grip of pain; we sit down on the threshold of God's purpose and die away of self-pity, and all so called Christian sympathy will aid us to our

death bed. But God will not. He comes with the grip of the pierced hand of His Son, and says—"Enter into fellowship with Me; arise and shine." If through a broken heart God can bring His purposes to pass in the world, then thank Him for breaking your heart.

The presence of the Holy Spirit saturated my spirit, soothing and healing the broken parts. I prayed, telling God that I was tired of taking Tim to doctors, that it had almost destroyed him, and that all I wanted was for Tim to be well. The darkness that had weighed me down diminished slowly. A renewed sense of peace and courage to go on, to face life, to believe that Tim and I both would some day be well, quietly filtered through me.

Later that morning I phoned Dr. Kenyon's office again, but it was his day off. I asked his secretary what decision the doctor had made. She said he had been swamped and was unable to call me. At this point I became exasperated. "Is the doctor even willing to talk to me?"

"Oh, yes," she assured me, "if you will call tomorrow at 1:30, he will talk to you."

14

The Diary

Dr. Kenyon finally agreed to change Tim's prescription and put him on Dilantin. He explained that it would take two or three weeks for it to saturate his system. Instinctively I felt that part of Tim's problem was an adverse reaction to the drug he was taking, and I hoped that the Dilantin, coupled with therapy, would diminish his disruptive behavior.

I recorded Tim's behavior during the transition from his previous medication to Dilantin. But it is a typical record of his actions and reactions at the peak of one of his electrical cycles.

Friday, November 2

A.M.—Excellent morning. Tim was happy, played with the dog, watched television.

3:50 P.M.

I'd been running errands. Arrived home half hour after Tim. Picked up Kevin and Tim. Left for cleaners and drugstore.

Tim told us, "I had a fight at school. And I ate ten pieces of candy before you got home."

At the cleaners, Kevin made a remark that caused me to respond jokingly, "You're a good kid."

Tim retorted, "You don't think I'm good, do you, because you make me take pills?"

Kevin: "If Mom and Dad didn't love you they wouldn't give you pills."

Discussion about therapy and pills followed.

At the drugstore, Tim announced, "I want these binoculars."

I reminded him, "You don't have any money. Maybe you can earn the money for them or work something out with Bill to earn them."

Tim became angry, and crushed the box with his fingers. I took the box away and returned it to toy counter.

A few minutes later, Tim picked the binoculars back up, followed me to the checkout stand, and plopped them on the counter. "You should buy me the binoculars because Kevin's buying a folder!" (The folder was for a science report.)

I took the binoculars away again, handed them to Kevin, who put them back. Tim became furious, gestured at me, and left the store. (*I thought*.)

I completed my purchases, walked out, sensed that Tim was behind me, and turned around.

Tim ran past me and out the door.

I grabbed his shirt in time to prevent him from running full force into an oncoming car.

Tim smacked the fender of the car with the flat of his hand. He leaped onto the hood of our car and refused to get off.

Finally I removed him bodily and put him in our car.

Tim ranted, cursed, and argued. He hit me on the back with both fists.

"Tim, if you don't stop, you'll have to go to bed at 7:00 P.M."

Kevin restrained Tim.

I repeated my early bedtime warning several more times.

Tim cried, screamed, and cursed. He ripped the cleaner bag

off the clothes. He broke away from Kevin, hurtled himself across the seat, grabbed Kevin's folder, and tried to rip it up.

Kevin subdued Tim just as we turned onto our street.

Ron's car was parked in the driveway.

"I'm running away from home!" Tim threatened. "And I'm going to tell Bill on you." He slung the car door open and charged down the street.

Ron: "Leave him where he is. He'll be all right."

I checked on Tim periodically. He played with his friends as if nothing had happened. I called him for dinner.

5:45 P.M.

Tim came home as if he'd never threatened to run away. He fussed at the dinner table. "You bought Kevin a folder," he reminded me. "You should've bought me the binoculars."

Ron and I explained why he couldn't have binoculars and why Kevin needed the folder.

Tim cursed.

Ron tried to kid Tim out of it.

Tim attacked Ron verbally and refused to respond. "Can I get out of going to bed early?" he asked.

"No," Ron and I replied.

Tim went to his room and screamed. "I'm gonna chop you so low an ant will walk on your umbrella!" He cried and ranted and raged. Then he turned on the radio full blast and started gyrating up and down in his room.

I went into his room, talked to him for a long time, got him to lie on the bed, and rubbed his back. After ten minutes I left the room.

Tim wept and wailed repeatedly, "I can't help myself! I can't help myself!" He finally quieted down after half an hour.

6:30 P.M.

I went in and asked, "Do you want to watch television?"

Tim: "No, I want to go to bed."

We talked awhile, prayed together, and I encouraged him to

see Ron.

Ron was deeply discouraged and depressed. (He doesn't become downhearted as easily as I do, but that evening he had one of his few times of self-searching.)

Tim and Ron talked until 7:00 P.M.

Tim went to bed.

Saturday, November 3

Early morning

Tim rose before all of us and ate a bunch of cookies (without permission). He watched television and played with the dog.

8:45 A.M.

Ron, Kevin, and I got up.

This was Tim's first day on Dilantin. Tim took a pill at 9:15 A.M. He repeatedly sang, "I need to jump, I need to jump," and gyrated wildly up—down—and around the room. He panted with his tongue hanging out like a dog, "Huhh-ahuhh-a-huhh."

"Get dressed!" I urged.

Tim kept parroting, "I need to jump," and ignored my request.

I took him by the arm, directed him to the bedroom, and reminded him, "You need to get dressed." I got his clothes out, handed them to him, and kept saying, "Put your clothes on." Finally I asked, "Is that the way you feel?"

"I have that jumpy feeling," Tim responded. After dressing, he calmed down, stopped what he was saying, and helped Kevin get the camping gear organized. Suddenly, however, he jumped up and down and pounded his bottom with clenched fists. He hit himself so hard, I was sure he'd bruise himself if I didn't stop him.

Finally he went outside and played with some friends. He came in at noon and asked to go with Russell to the park. He was away the rest of the day with Russell's family. He enjoyed his day.

He had a good evening.

Sunday, November 4

Tim was upset. Kevin was home sick with the flu and didn't go to church. Tim expressed anger, but went to church without being unduly upset.

An excellent day. Ron and Tim ate lunch out and went fishing.

Very good evening.

Monday, November 5

Excellent morning.

Tim took a shower on his own. "Some physical fitness dudes are coming to my school," he explained. "I don't want them to see me dirty." He talked a while in repetitious lisp talk.

After school, we had an appointment with Bill.

Tim did not become overly upset with me when I couldn't say, "You haven't argued."

Excellent afternoon and evening.

Tuesday, November 6

Happy morning.

Tim hummed songs, teased, and laughed. He was less intense when he woke up, with less lisp and less talking through clenched teeth since going on Dilantin.

"I threw candy in the lunchroom yesterday," Tim confessed before leaving. "I'll have to stay after school for an hour." Then he told me about a fight he'd had at school.

3:10 P.M.

Tim came home on time. "The teacher didn't get the note from the lunchroom monitor," Tim announced. "I didn't have to stay after school. Can I have a malt?"

"You can have one with dinner," I told him.

"Then I'll eat a bunch of my Halloween candy," Tim said angrily as he helped himself to some candy. Tim told the dog when he let him in, "Now don't you be hypergenic [his word for hyperactive]. Lick me but don't bite me!"

Tim talked to the dog, pulling the animal up by its front paws. "Me and Simba jump," he explained as he started jumping around the room with the dog.

Kevin became keyed up, pushed Tim to stop him, and pretended to do Kung-Fu on Tim.

Tim yelled, "I need to jump! I want to jump!"

I broke the fight up and told them, "Think of something else to do."

"Let's take the dog for a walk," Kevin suggested. They left.

Before supper

"Guess what I am in the classroom?" Tim asked.

I couldn't guess.

Tim made me guess several times. Finally he announced, "I was voted vice-president of my class. A girl and I ran, and she only got five votes. All the guys came around and asked me, 'What does it feel like to be vice-president?' "

"What are you going to do as vice-president?" I asked.

"Take care of the calendar, and take the place of the president when he's absent."

My diary writing suffered when a dish and bed breaking binge broke out in our house after dinner.

Simba put his paws on the sink top. He tried to lick any leftovers out of the dishes and a drinking cup fell to the floor. Splinters of glass splattered everywhere.

While Kevin was slushing soapsuds over a sink full of dirty dishes, he stuck his hand in a glass and broke it.

Before bedtime Ron was peacefully reading the newspaper on our bed. Kevin and Tim decided to join him. Because there wasn't enough room, Kevin shoved Tim with his foot and Tim pushed back. I was reading when I heard a crack—crack—whoom—whoosh and crumble!

"Ha—ha—ha—ha!" Tim laughed hysterically. "The bed

broke. We're too fat. Ha—ha—ha! We're all too fat!"

"If you hadn't been wrestling each other, the bed wouldn't have broken," Ron grumbled.

Tim stood over the crumpled shambles and continued to laugh uncontrollably. Kevin and I giggled but tried not to laugh out loud. Ron didn't think it was humorous.

"I don't think this is funny at all!" Ron announced indignantly. "We'll have to buy a new frame and sleep on the floor until we get one."

Tim laughed so hard he almost cried. Kevin and I continued to snicker while we helped clean up the crumbled debris.

"What's so hilarious? I don't think it's funny at all!" Ron snorted.

Wednesday, November 7

Tim topped off the breaking brigade the next morning. He was opening a can of food for the dog and hit a bowl with his hand; it slipped and shattered all over.

"Well, Tim," I laughed, "we're on a breaking binge—two glasses, a bowl, and a bed."

"That was so funny last night when the bed broke." Tim giggled.

After school

I went with Tim to the junior high to watch Kevin play in a football game. Kevin's team won 30-6.

7:00 P.M.

Tim had another "I need to jump" spell. I informed him, "You'll have to go to your room if you're going to jump, or find something else to do." So he went to Brian's and played at his house for an hour.

Good evening.

Thursday, November 8
Morning

Tim was tired and had a hard time getting going. He became stimulated. "I need to jump," he said.

"We should talk to Bill about your need to jump," I told him. "You need to break yourself of it."

Tim's eyes widened. "You wouldn't tell Bill. You'd be embarrassed."

"I think you need to work on it, don't you?"

Tim didn't answer. He went to his room.

3:15 P.M.

Tim mowed the lawn.

4:30 P.M.

I decided to go grocery shopping.

"I want to go along!" Tim shouted.

"It's Kevin's turn. You can go the next time," I explained. (I usually take either Kevin or Tim so I can have time alone with each one.)

Tim got mad and started to argue.

"It's Kevin's turn," I repeated. "You can go next time. What flavor of ice cream would you like me to buy?"

"Chocolate chip," Tim said.

I started to drive out of the driveway but had to return. I had forgotten my grocery list.

Tim draped himself over a fender of the car and cursed. Finally he got off, but ran back and forth behind the car in the street.

Ron came out.

Tim ran away, cursing and gesturing wildly as we drove down the street.

"I don't understand it," I said, perplexed. "Tim had an excellent morning."

"When he has a good morning, he has rotten days and when he has rotten mornings, he has good days," Kevin said. "Yesterday, Tim was in a fight with Raymond and pounded him pretty hard. It really scared me because Tim hurt Raymond."

"Why didn't you break it up?" I questioned.

"I tried, but I couldn't stop him. I tried to tell Raymond's mother that Tim was hypo. [The true definition of "hypo" is underactive.] She said, 'Hypo, hell; let them fight it out.' But Tim really snuffed Raymond." (Kevin was visibly shaken just recalling the incident.)

Dinner table

Tim didn't like dinner and was mad. (He'd requested the menu the night before.)

Ron and I both reminded him, "This was the dinner you requested last night."

Tim tore at his food with his fork as he ate. "You brought the wrong kind of ice cream," he announced. "And the *next time* you go to the store, it's *my* turn!"

Evening

Tim watched television, cleaned his room, sat on our bed with Kevin, and read the Sears toy catalog for a long time.

Friday, November 9

Morning

"I'm not going to school," Tim declared.

"Fine! You may stay home," I told him. "But you will go to bed at six o'clock tonight!"

Tim argued.

"I won't discuss it," I said flatly. I took a shower and refused to answer Tim.

Tim badgered me with argumentative declarations. He slugged the bathroom door with his fist.

Later Tim announced, "I ate my breakfast. I'm going to school." His pills were still on the table.

"Take your pills before you leave," I reminded him.

"I'm not going to take my pills," he said flatly. "I'll take my hypo-pill but not my vitamins."

"Why not the vitamins?"

"I take more pills than you do," Tim argued.

"Count them!" I countered.

Tim counted my vitamins, then his. We found that we took the same amount. He gulped his down with his milk. "I'm still hungry. I want my breakfast."

"Whose bowl is that on the table?" I shouted angrily.

"Kevin's."

"What do you want for breakfast?"

Tim giggled, "I already ate." He finished dressing, collected his books, and went out the door singing—but he was probably late for school.

3:10 P.M.

Tim didn't like my choice of snacks. "What's there to eat?" he griped. "There's nothing but crap in this house to eat!"

I made at least seven suggestions.

Tim rejected them all!

I refused to give him a bag of school lunch chips he requested. He fussed that any other foods were unacceptable. Finally he decided what he wanted and gulped it down.

He called David and asked if he could come over for the night.

I drove him to David's house.

On the way, Tim remarked, "You make me hypergenic!"

"How do I make you hypergenic?" I asked, surprised by the statement.

"When you yell at me."

"How do you think I feel when you scream at me?"

Tim laughed. "Hypergenic!"

Saturday, November 10

1:00 P.M.

Ron picked up Tim and David. They had planned a backpack trip to a regional park.

Tim had another "I-need-to-jump" spell. He lisped the same phrase over and over for twenty minutes while getting ready to go. The trip was successful. Tim carried his pack up and down the steep hills.

Excellent evening.

Sunday, November 11
Before church

Tim was nervous and keyed up. He twirled his fingers, jumped, and talked nonstop. I wanted to stay home. (I was sick.) Tim stalled long enough so Ron had to leave. He brought Simba in. The dog ran in circles.

Tim grabbed the collar and shook his finger at the dog. "Now don't you be hypergenic. We're going to make you a goof chart."

Simba chewed on Tim's arm.

Tim flared up. He threw the dog around and kicked at him. The dog ran in circles and scooted around, trying to stay out of Tim's way.

I put the dog outside.

Tim lay on the couch, his feet twitching. Suddenly he jumped up, went to the double glass doors, clenched his teeth, and lisped to the dog, "You stop being a bad boy. You're hypergenic. Now you just stop, you dumb dog." Tim pressed his face against the glass and repeated his lisped warnings to dog.

I gave Tim ideas of things he could do.

Excellent afternoon and evening.

Monday, November 12
Before school

Tim was keyed up and nervous again. His fingers twitched. He talked constantly and acted silly, embarrassing Kevin.

"Go to your room until Kevin leaves for school," Ron told him.

After Kevin left, Tim was in an "I-need-to-jump" mood again. He sang a song about jumping that he made up and then got into another wild wrestling match with the dog. I put the dog out. Neither Tim nor the dog would settle down.

3:10 P.M.

I picked Tim up at school. We had another appointment with Bill.

"How have I done this week?" Tim asked. "I socked a boy so hard in the mouth that his lip bled," Tim bantered on. "The teacher sent me to the principal." (The story later turned out to be untrue.) "How have I done this week?" Tim kept asking.

"I honestly can't say you've controlled yourself," I told him.

Tim became hostile and rebelled against going in for more therapy. He wanted to earn points and knew he couldn't. He threw himself all over the office rug and couch.

After the therapy session with Bill, Tim was angry. "Bill took away ten points for the way I acted up." (The loss of ten points also proved to be untrue.)

Tim settled down at home and was fine the rest of the evening.

10:00 P.M.

I arrived home from the meeting. Ron and Kevin were asleep.

Tim called, "Mom, will you pray with me?"

Tim prayed: "Dear Lord, please help Walt with his asthma. Help me so I won't have temper tantrums anymore, and that I won't do bad things. Amen."

Tuesday, November 13

Early morning

Tim is not as crabby as he was when he was taking the other drug. But his hands twist, twitch, and turn a lot. He talks nonstop. This morning he is in a good mood. He started to talk about jumping.

I sent him to his room for five minutes.

Tim kept yelling over and over, "How many more minutes?" When the time was up, he took a shower. (It's picture day at school.) After the shower he talked about jumping again.

"You'll go back to your room," I warned.

Tim stopped. His hair was sopping wet. He wanted me to use the hair dryer on his hair. He sat on the footstool for ten minutes while I blew warm air over his hair with a wand. The whirring sound and warmth seemed to mesmerize him. He has been more cheerful, less depressed and groggy.

3:15 P.M.

Kevin was baking a cake when Tim came home.

Tim got mad. "I've never made a cake before." (He makes cookies all the time.) Tim watched Kevin and refused to do his own chores. He repeatedly sneaked back into the kitchen. He told Kevin throughout the entire cake and frosting process, "It's a crap cake!"

Kevin became agitated at Tim's remarks about the "crap cake." Kevin knocked Tim around in a wrestling match outside. They broke the fight up themselves, but continued to take verbal potshots at each other.

Evening

Both boys settled down and watched television. Tim ate two pieces of the "crap cake," as he continued to refer to it, and wanted more.

Wednesday, November 14

Outstanding morning.

Tim was in an excellent mood. He wasn't nervous.

After school

Tim was in a happy mood.

Keyed up, Kevin pushed, poked, and wrestled with Tim. Tim didn't become angry. He just giggled and laughed.

Thursday, November 15

Another excellent morning.

Tim didn't have mood swings, lethargy, or need to "jump." The Dilantin seems to be taking hold. Tim's more alert both morning and evening. He doesn't require as much sleep and is not as intense.

Later he confessed, "Last night when I was supposed to be in the junior class at church, I stayed out and told everyone who asked that I was sick."

3:10 P.M.

Tim came home from school in a good mood. But he asked Kevin to come into the bedroom because he had a secret to tell him.

Kevin told me later, "Tim wanted me to beat up a boy who had been picking fights with him on the way home from school."

Tim did yard work. Then he packed clothes for a weekend at Green Oak Boys Ranch.

Excellent evening.

Friday, November 16

Very good morning.

Tim said, "Let's jump. No, I'm sorry." He never repeated it again. Instead of saying, "I need to jump," he sang in singsong tones, "Aye—yee—yee! Viva! Viva! Aye—yee—yee! Viva! Viva!" at least eighty times. I think he has a broken record syndrome. The number of times he repeats a favored phrase is incredible. He drove me to distraction with his endless refrain. But he was happy, cheerful, and fairly calm despite it. And he talked a lot.

I told him, "You've had a better week."

"I don't have to worry, because I'll be at camp. All I have left is to earn points on Monday, because I'll be gone." (He was to see Bill on Monday.)

After school

Tim was excited about camp. He flitted from one thing to the next, but finally organized himself.

5:00 P.M.

Tim left for camp with the church gang on a bus. It was a cold, crisp night and rain was predicted.

In retrospect we know that the drug Tim took prior to Dilantin intensified his behavior in a bizarre manner. He was on that drug two times for nine months. Both times it built up in his system and affected him detrimentally. Unfortunately, this is only one of the many adverse complexities of the prescribed drug world. Dilantin proved to be what Tim needed.

15

Paradox

Rain stampeded in on Saturday. I could envision Tim wound up and wild because he was confined to the camp buildings. I could also picture him sloshing in the mud, riding the horses, and playing outside despite the downpour.

Sunday afternoon Tim arrived home in the condition of my second vision. His voice was froggy and he could hardly croak out his words. His hair looked like a dirty dishrag, his blue clothes were stiff with muck, and his face and arms were as grubby as the rest of him.

He dumped out a suitcase full of wet, smelly clothes and treasures. Proudly he showed us a wood picture he'd made with a real horseshoe mounted on it. He croaked out his stories a mile-a-minute and told us about his slushy hikes, donkey rides, and games in the mud.

He confessed that he acted up in chapel. "I couldn't sit still and the sheriff took me out of the meeting. When he asked me my name, I told him, 'Joe Mack Cragg.'

"When we were getting ready to leave, the sheriff wanted to know if we wanted to take a Bible study. He asked me, 'Joe, would you like one?' " Tim howled. "I fooled him. I fooled him. He thought my name was Joe." The highlight of Tim's weekend at camp was telling everyone the story of how he fooled the sheriff.

Tim took a shower and went to bed early—exhilarated, exhausted, and proclaiming that he wanted to go back to camp next week.

The following weekend was the Thanksgiving holiday. Friday, Ron rose early to attend a men's prayer breakfast. I slept late. Kevin and Tim woke me by flopping on my bed. We were laughing and reminiscing when Tim fussed, "I itch!" He pulled up his T-shirt and showed me a rash. He was covered from his neck to his toes.

"How long have you had this?" I gasped.

"Since Wednesday," he answered nonchalantly.

"Oh, no! Tim! You exposed the kids at school, the people at Thanksgiving service at church, and the rest of our family yesterday. Why didn't you tell me?" I moaned.

Tim wasn't sure why he hadn't thought to tell me. All I could think of was the number of people who would have to be informed that they'd been exposed to measles.

The earliest doctor's appointment we could obtain was at 3:45 P.M. Tim had to stay in the house all day. He was nervous and kept asking, "Do I have to have a shot?" I didn't think he would need one, but I couldn't convince him of that.

When Dr. Kenyon saw the rash, he immediately said, "Tim doesn't have the measles. This is an allergic reaction to the Dilantin. You'll have to take Tim off the Dilantin for four days, and then try again. If he still has a reaction, we'll have to find something else to give him. I'll prescribe some medicine to stop the itching."

When I told Ron that evening about our dilemma, he was concerned, because he would be leaving on Sunday for a tour of his company plant in Ohio. He would be gone a week, and he knew Tim would spiral without something to calm him down.

By the following Monday Tim began to show signs that he hadn't had his Dilantin. He couldn't concentrate on television. His arms, body, and legs jerked and moved like a movie sped up to double-time. First it was a drink of water, then a piece of cake, then an apple, then outside—back inside—outside gain, on the couch and off, twisting, turning, moving every few minutes.

It was 10:30 before I finally got him settled for bed. He asked me to pray with him.

"Dear Jesus," he prayed, "thank you for the good day today. Help me not to be hypergenic. Watch over my dad in Idaho—Ohio. Watch over my dog. Watch over the Taylors. Watch over Eric and Rod, and help Walt with his asthma. Amen."

The next afternoon after school I took Tim and Kevin with me to do several errands, one of which was to buy some parts for Kevin's newly acquired used electric train set. Tim became angry on our way to the train shop because I was doing something for Kevin and not for him, even though Kevin was spending money he had earned himself. Tim didn't know what he wanted, but he was still mad. I started to explain. Before I knew it we were arguing. I realized we were riding on the merry-argue-go-round again; I needed to stop and get off.

"Tim, I'm not going to argue with you. The discussion is over. I'll talk with you about anything else, but I won't argue."

"I can't talk then, can I?" he snapped back.

"Yes, you can talk," I countered, "but I won't argue."

"I can't talk. I can't talk. I can't talk," he parroted.

Suddenly he stopped talking and refused to say another word. For the next two hours he showed us what he wanted by making motions with his hands.

Although Tim refused to talk he kept bugging Kevin while he tried to set up the train track. The train-track connections kept shorting out and Kevin couldn't get his electric train running.

Tim stood at the sidelines and laughed in mocking silence every time Kevin had trouble. Kevin's natural abilities and the ease with which he accomplishes projects frustrates Tim and makes him feel inferior. And so Tim's target for taunting is Kevin. Every time I caught Tim bothering Kevin I sent him somewhere else, but he continued to sneak into the garage where Kevin was working.

In return Kevin pounded and punched Tim even when Tim wasn't bothering him. Later that evening before bed Kevin deliberately opened a Christmas gift Tim had made for us. It was Kevin's way of getting back at Tim.

When I bawled Kevin out he began to cry. I made Tim go to bed, shut the bedroom door, and brought Kevin out to the living room where we could talk.

I told Kevin, "You're wrecking things. We're trying to help Tim and yet you've been hitting him and punching him every chance you get."

"I'm sick of helping him," Kevin sobbed. "I don't want to help him anymore. What good does it do? Nothing changes."

I wrapped my arms around Kevin. "Kevin, we love you and appreciate you. It gets to us, too, when Tim acts the way he does. But when your dad's gone, it's even harder. Tim misses Dad and acts up worse. We're taking him to therapy to try to help him."

"He's still the same. Therapy doesn't help." Kevin wept and poured out his feelings.

Kevin then admitted that he was jealous of Tim. We had denied our own rights to meet Tim's needs. Tears streamed down our cheeks. I held Kevin in my arms and we sat in silence for a long time. Both of us were drained.

We'd placed too much of the burden of control on Ron, Kevin, and me. It wasn't that we didn't discipline Tim, because we did. But he couldn't clearly understand the consequences of his actions, nor differentiate between right and wrong, what was harmful and what was not.

Ron and I had to teach Tim the simple values of the rights

of others and family relationships. And the only way we seemed to reach Tim was to be completely calm and self-controlled at all times.

Many times though, Tim *did* understand and he manipulated us by acting like he didn't know what we were talking about. It was a constant judgment battle for us. "Is this something he doesn't understand? Or is he just manipulating us again?"

Some of Tim's angry outbursts, hostility, irritability, and tantrums were acts of frustrated fury at our controlling—preventing—stopping and restricting his acts of poor judgment. Other times the buildup of electricity seemed to switch on and light up rage from seemingly insignificant, minor occurrences that had nothing to do with us.

When Tim woke up Thursday morning he was in a cheerful mood. At breakfast he remembered, "Oh, I almost forgot. This is the day I'm supposed to start taking my pill again."

"That's right!" I was surprised. Tim resented taking his pills.

"I feel like I need it," he stated quietly.

Later I opened the back door so I could feed Simba. He charged past me, slid across the floor, shook, wiggled, then jumped all over me.

Simba ran around investigating everything, stopping only to lick up cereal crumbs under Tim's chair. I started toward the bedroom. Then a mass of brown fur whizzed by me and flew onto Tim's unmade bed. Four black paw prints stamped their indelible marks on the white bed sheets.

Simba stopped to scratch, then scrambled onto Kevin's bed autographing more sheets with his paws. Suddenly, Simba swooped up Tim's cinnamon brown teddy bear and shook it vigorously.

Tim pushed Simba on his side and held him down with both hands. In his clenched-teeth lisp he scolded the dog. "You bad dog. Give me back my bear." Tim pried open Simba's mouth and retrieved the bear. "Now calm down and behave yourself.

Leave my bear alone. Just stop being hypergenic." Tim scolded, wagging the bear in Simba's face.

"Let the dog go and get him off the bed," I urged.

Tim pulled Simba off the bed and the dog scrambled into the other room. "Mom. Do you think there'll be dogs in heaven?" he asked unexpectedly.

"There might be," I replied. "God created all the animals and dogs."

"*I love dogs!* Do you really think there will be?"

"There might be, son."

"I sure hope so!"

"Well, maybe you can become a keeper of animals in heaven," I teased.

"I'm going to give my brown bear to Simba," Tim announced, changing the subject. "Every time he comes into my room, he grabs one of my bears."

I laughed. "Yes, his favorite toys do seem to be your teddy bears. Finish dressing now. I have to make your lunch."

As I entered the kitchen I heard a "slurp—slurp—slurp." Simba had his paws hooked over the top edge of the sink. His head lay sideways over a bowl of leftover cereal. His long tongue stretched to reach inside the bowl, so he could lap up the milk. Milk and cereal splattered all over the sink and floor. String of shredded cereal plastered Simba's face, chest, ears, and head. I scolded Simba and pushed his paws off the counter.

Tim had followed me and we both broke out laughing. Simba cocked his head. His big brown eyes seemed to say, "What's so funny?"

Tim still had his bear in his hand and shook it at the dog. "You stop being a bad boy." Tim knelt down and grabbed Simba's collar. "You can have this bear. You leave my other bear alone! You're going outside, Hypergenic!" Tim dragged the dog out the door.

Tim and I stood at the double-glass doors and watched Simba sprint around the yard. The bear dangled and flopped helplessly out of his mouth. For a second Simba stopped and snapped the bear from side to side. Then he raced round and round the track he'd worn in our yard.

On Sunday after Ron got home we started a new game to help Tim sit still, listen, and endure the church services. For a thousand points he could earn a trip to his favorite ice cream parlor. Both of our pastors print their sermons. We picked out the main words, and wrote them on a separate piece of paper. Every time Tim heard one of the words he would put a mark by it. We would count the number of marks he made and that's how many points he'd earn during the service. At the close Tim remarked, "Boy, church went by fast. It wasn't boring."

Monday, Mrs. Davis phoned to say, "I would like to place Tim in a special physical education program. He refuses to cooperate during regular physical education. He seems to lack coordination in most of the games that require fine muscle movements and skill.

"The only game he isn't frustrated by is football. I'm sending home a permission slip. Would you please sign it and send it back right away?"

"Sure, that's fine with us. How's he doing in class?"

"Well," she paused. "He's been in a few fights. And he's farther behind in his work."

"Could we have a conference?"

"How about tomorrow afternoon right after school?"

Tuesday afternoon when I walked past the school office to Tim's classroom, he came out. I gasped. Tim's mouth was bleeding. His tooth had been knocked out and he was crying, "Gene beat me up," he stammered. "My teacher didn't do a thing about it!"

Just then Mrs. Davis appeared and she proceeded to tell the other side of the story. "Tim has been threatening Gene every day for the past few weeks. He kept telling Gene, 'I'm going to get my big brother at junior high school to beat you up.' Gene is the kind of kid that you don't push around. Gene finally had enough and popped Tim in the mouth."

Tim was mad and tried to quarrel with Mrs. Davis. Before he could get started, I sent him home so we could have our conference.

"Tim is so different from last year," Mrs. Davis began. "I just can't get over the change in him. He was so cooperative last year, but now he's belligerent. He fights, and today he refused to sing with the kids who were practicing the school Christmas program. He's doing third-grade work, which makes him considerably behind."

"And he's supposed to be in the fifth grade."

Tears welled up in her eyes when she wistfully answered, "The other kids are beginning to laugh at Tim because he doesn't understand simple directions."

"He needs to be in a learning disability class then, doesn't he?"

"Yes, but the waiting list is long," she sighed. "I just had a boy transfer into my class that needs a full day in a class for the emotionally handicapped. I have several other children that need a class as much or more than Tim does. I doubt if he can get into a class until next year, and maybe not then."

I slumped in my chair. I was sick. Tim had the finest of teachers and even that was not enough. The pressure-cooker stress of not understanding instructions and being behind was too much for Tim.

I hurried away from our meeting because Tim had an appointment with Bill. At the end of Tim's session, he came out proudly carrying a foam Nerf football he'd earned by cooperating in his weekly sessions.

All the rest of the week Tim carried his football everywhere. Tuesday, in the middle of the night, Tim climbed out of bed while still asleep and shook Kevin with both hands. "Give me my Nerf ball. Give me back my Nerf ball." Then Tim tried to get into Kevin's bed.

Kevin called for Ron. "Daddy, Tim's in bed with me." Ron got up, walked Tim back to his bed, covered him up, and Tim never knew the difference.

Every day after school Tim played Nerf ball with Simba. Tim threw the ball. Simba leaped through the air, caught it between his teeth, then raced around the yard with Tim in pursuit. Suddenly Simba screeched to a halt, dropped the ball, and waited for Tim to creep up on him. Just as Tim grabbed for the ball, Simba snapped it up and scooted off.

One day a week later, Simba sneaked the beige bear and chewed several chunks out of the foam football. Tim was so irate he screamed, "You bad dog! Look at what you did to my ball. And you bit holes in my bear. You have your own bear. You bad dog!"

Tim pummeled, punched and pushed the dog with his fists and feet. "Yipe! Yipe! Yipe!" Simba yowled.

I heard the commotion in time to stop Tim from hurting the dog. I put Simba outside. The cinnamon brown bear lay dusty and dirty, teeth punctured and torn under the apricot tree, with only its head, arm, and half a body still intact. Simba snatched the bear up, shook it, then raced around the yard.

I sent Tim to his room for a long time-out. The last few weeks we'd clamped a tight lid on Tim. We'd made it clear that he was responsible for his actions and that he could and would have to learn to control and contain himself.

Stark reality, however, blew dark clouds into our life. Intermittent rainstorms of problems had fallen in the past at school, but now we were faced with a thunderstorm. Mrs. Davis had continued to keep us posted. Before we had experienced many cooperative, productive, sunshine days with Tim—mixed with some stormy behavior. But a steady, swift torrent of fighting, refusing to participate, not paying attention, not completing work, and hostility now flooded Tim's days.

We honestly wondered if we were making a serious mistake. We had not anticipated Tim's role reversal. We were perplexed at his paradoxical personality. How could he remain in control of himself, charming and delightful, and then suddenly switch into a fit of oppositional fury?

Mrs. Davis was an outstanding teacher. We knew it had

nothing to do with her. She was tired and I was sure she looked forward to the coming Christmas vacation.

The last week of school before vacation, Tim asked, "Can I buy a Christmas gift for my teacher?" When I took him to the store, he picked out a card with a sentimental, affectionate verse "For Teacher." The gift-selecting decision was not so easy. Tim had expensive tastes and it took him a long time to settle on a box of scented soaps.

At home when he started to fill out the card he asked hesitantly, "Another girl put 'God bless you' on her card. Do you think I should write, 'May God be with you'?"

"Sure, if you want to. I think your teacher would like that."

Tim wrote the words on his card, then added, "Love, Tim." He licked the gummed seal on the envelope, pressed it down tightly, put the card under the lid of the box, then started to wrap the Christmas paper around it. "Wait a minute," I blurted, "you're supposed to put the card on the outside of the box after you wrap it."

Tim snickered, shrugged his shoulders, and sheepishly admitted, "I don't want anyone to see what I wrote. They'll laugh at me."

16

No Easy Answers, No Miracle Cures

Christmas vacation began later than usual. It was only four days until Christmas. Sunday morning, December 23, I woke up at 5:00. My body was fighting another bladder infection and I had the chills. Three days prior, my left knee had begun to ache. I thought I had a catch in it, that I could walk it out and the pain would go away. Instead, my knee ached and throbbed intensely and I couldn't sleep.

I thought I'd slip out of bed and lie by the living room heater. I tried to inch my way out of bed so I wouldn't wake Ron. He's sensitive to noise and always knows when I've been sick or had a rough night. He'd been losing enough sleep himself and had been so concerned that I didn't want to disturb him.

Surging waves of nausea ebbed and flowed through me. I tried to make it to the bathroom. Instead I slid down the hall wall and passed out. A few seconds later I came to and barely made it back to bed before I blacked out again. Ron woke up.

Around 8:00 A.M. Ron decided that I was going to the hospital. I kept insisting, "My knee will be okay. Remember when I did this once before and in a few days I walked it out?"

Ron examined my swollen knee and adamantly announced, "You're going to the hospital!"

I kept thinking, "The doctor will put an elastic bandage on my knee and send me home." I was shocked when he diagnosed the injury as a torn knee cartilage. The doctor chuckled when he informed me that the injury was common among football players. "You haven't been playing any football lately, have you?" he teased.

I didn't think it was so humorous; I couldn't even remember twisting my knee and had no idea how or when it was injured. With the exception of doing a few household chores, I'd been pretty inactive because I'd been so ill.

The doctor said he was going to wrap my leg in an elastic plaster bandage, from my ankle to the top of my thigh. He then informed me I would have to stay off my leg. The cast would be removed in two weeks so he could recheck my knee.

Christmas morning Tim woke up about 5:30. I don't believe he would have awakened so early, except the engine of a truck parked in the next door driveway closest to our bedrooms rumbled, reverberated, and rattled our windows for twenty minutes or more. Ron finally relented at 6:00 and let the boys get up to open the small gifts in their stockings.

At 6:30 Ron and I couldn't withstand Tim's early morning excitement any longer. We crawled and hobbled out of bed. Ron suggested that we open our Christmas celebration with prayer.

Both boys tried to disguise their disappointment. Ron knew they would rather put off praying; present opening had been prolonged long enough. "I'm going to preach a long sermon," Ron teased. "Now, Tim, don't you call anything I say boring." He waved his arms in the air, pretending to preach a sermon, and we all laughed.

After we settled down we bowed our heads and Ron led us in a prayer of thanksgiving for all that God had provided through the gift of His Son and through the gifts we were able to give in remembrance of this event.

One at a time Ron passed gifts to Kevin and Tim. Then we waited to see what was in each package before Ron handed out another one. One huge package for Tim intrigued the boys.

Ron finally dramatically ushered the boys over to the large box. Tim tore at the paper, throwing and shredding it as he pulled it off the box. "An organ!" he exclaimed.

We had bought him a small chord organ. Tim has always loved music, and we hoped this would be something he could learn to play and enjoy. Immediately he was able to figure out how to read the numbered songbooks and to play the organ. The rest of the day the organ took center stage.

All of us had to try our hand at it. But Tim seemed to have a natural sense of rhythm, and although he had never played anything before, the music flowed through his fingers with feeling and proper timing.

On December 31 I had an appointment with Dr. Campbell. I was to have a hysterectomy in January, but Dr. Campbell took one look at my cast-covered leg and said matter-of-factly, "I'm afraid the surgery will have to be postponed indefinitely. If you're going to need knee surgery, that will have to come first. You have to be free to move around without a cast or crutches following a hysterectomy."

The shock of postponing the surgery was almost unbearable. I didn't want to face having pain and taking medication for it for an undetermined length of time.

I tried to believe that this was what God felt was best, but could not help questioning everything we were facing as a family. I longed for a miracle cure and was not sure I could endure this time of intense testing. A feeling of despair depressed me, and the will to face life bravely slipped silently from me.

Tim had gone to stay with the Taylors for a couple of days. Tim is sensitive to me, and my present state of emotional instability would have triggered him and shot him into his own imbalanced upheaval.

Tim's absence gave me time to retreat, to regroup my thinking, and to regain my inner strength. I took the opportunity that the quiet afforded to search the Scriptures and set down some thoughts for the New Year. God's Word had spoken directly to my needs many times before, and I hoped to find something to hold on to, a sense of security in God's care and concern for my family and me, and most of all, a renewed will to go on.

The words that Paul had written regarding his physical affliction drew me, and I knew that they were there for me at that moment.

> And so, to keep me from being unduly elated by the magnificence of such revelations, I was given a sharp physical pain which came as Satan's messenger to bruise me; this was to save me from being unduly elated. Three times I begged the Lord to rid me of it [Oh how many times I had prayed this prayer with Paul], but his answer was: *"My grace is all you need; power comes to its full strength in weakness."* I shall therefore prefer to find my joy and pride in the very things that are my weakness; and then the power of Christ will come and rest upon me. Hence I am well content, for Christ's sake, with weakness . . . hardship, and frustration; for when I am weak, then I am strong (2 Cor. 12:7-10, italics added).
>
> What then? I will pray as I am inspired to pray, but I will also pray intelligently. I will sing hymns as I am inspired to sing, but I will sing intelligently too (1 Cor. 14:15).
>
> Christ is all that matters, for Christ lives in . . . all (Col. 3:11, *Phillips*).

Then I took a printed card out of a box of quotations and single Scriptures to mark my place in my Bible for devotions, "He that shall humble himself shall be exalted," Matthew 23:12.

On the reverse side of the card was a quotation by Abraham Lincoln. "I have been driven many times to my knees, by the overwhelming conviction that I had nowhere else to go. My own wisdom, and that of all about me, seemed insufficient for that day."

The words ministered to me. The unity of thoughts from Scripture and the quote renewed my courage.

Tim returned home late in the afternoon of New Year's Day. Although he and David had had a great time, Tim was hostile that afternoon and the next two days. He refused to clean up any of the messes he made. When he played with Kevin's Christmas games, he'd leave them lay. "They're not mine," he explained and took off outside. He demanded I do things he knew I couldn't do. "You're faking it! There's nothing the matter with your leg. You do it!"

He became even more belligerent when I refused to comply with his commands. Confining him to his room for brief periods of punishment and threatening that he'd lose points when he saw Bill didn't work. An I-don't-care-what-you-do-to-me attitude prevailed.

By Wednesday Kevin and I both had had it and we blew up and exploded at Tim most of the day. At 6:30 that evening we had an appointment with Bill. I told him how impossible Tim had been since coming home from the Taylors.

"If Tim doesn't improve, maybe we should consider admitting him to a hospital for therapy," Bill suggested gently. "I know of an excellent hospital that specializes in working with children."

While Bill went on talking, a sense of numbness slowly came over me and all I could do was nod my head; I was too shaken.

I didn't say anything to Ron. He wasn't sure that therapy was making a difference. Tim was no better and he opposed therapy so much that Ron was ready to give up.

The next morning the weight of my sorrow and grief almost crushed me. Bill's remark about committing Tim to a psychiatric hospital was unbearable to me.

I forced myself to pick up my Bible, to have my devotions, and pray. The words were reaching out to me, but I still felt a deep sense of sorrow.

A few minutes after I finished reading, Pastor Carlson phoned to see how I was doing. He checked with us periodically and I was grateful to hear his voice. After I shared our latest concern, he prayed with me. God knew how much I needed to hear from someone.

A few minutes after talking with Pastor Carlson I talked at length with my closest friend, Leona. Her wisdom and ability to counsel have always been a special talent that God has given her. I knew God was using her to lift me out of the mire of depression.

Our mail arrived early. An unexpected letter from Edith, another friend, greeted me. We had not lived near each other for ten years, and it had been three years since I had last seen her. She was a special education teacher, and I had written to tell her about Tim and ask her advice. When her oldest boy was a toddler, I'd taken care of him often, and he missed me when we moved away.

She told me what kind of mother I had been to her own son, with Kevin, and other children. She was sure that Tim was probably doing much better because of the kind of person she remembered me to be. She closed by saying how much she still missed my friendship. Tears brimmed from my eyes. It touched me to think that even through a letter, on the day I imagined myself to be a failure as a mother, God sent His love and assurance.

God's special interest in my life amazed me. I began to catch a glimmer of hope and renewed feeling that He was working things out despite the circumstances.

Friday, January 12, sheets of silvery rain slipped across the grass. Yards of liquid slithered down the gutterless street. It was the first week of school following the Christmas and New Year's holidays. Although the downpour had turned to a drizzle, Tim was soaked when he arrived home.

After he changed, I went to put his wet clothes away and pulled two papers from his pants. Carefully I separated each one and laid them on the table to dry. I couldn't help but see a big *F* on each English paper.

After dinner that evening, Ron seemed disturbed. He slammed and banged things around, then griped about a television program I was watching.

When he finished his reports for work, he went to bed at 9:30. The boys were already in bed, so I turned off the television and followed.

"Something is really bothering you," I quietly murmured.

"It's Tim," he sighed.

"What's the matter?"

"His paper—he brought home. He's failing."

"I know," I said simply. "It doesn't seem fair that he should have to fail before he can get help."

"He's probably not the only one. They have many other children like Tim and the schools are short on funds. The school enrollment has been dropping. With fewer children maybe they'll be able to afford to do more," Ron reflected.

"The teacher told me that there are a lot of other children like Tim whose parents want help as much as we do."

Close to each other we lay quiet and still. Our hearts and minds—thinking, throbbing, touching—echoed in the silence.

"Sometimes there are no answers—are there? No easy answers," I whispered, breaking the silence.

"No—no there aren't!"

17

Love Is Not Enough

Almost every day Tim reminded me that January 22 was dog license day. Simba was old enough to have his first rabies and distemper shots. A city-wide campaign was underway to provide shots at a minimal fee and to license dogs.

For the first time Tim mentioned Rags. "I was so sad when Rags died. I don't want that to happen to Simba. If Simba has a license and he gets lost, then we can get him back. Can't we?"

"Yes, that's why we get a license."

"I missed Rags so much. And I don't want anything to happen to Simba."

"Do you remember what you did when Rags died?" I asked softly.

"I laughed," he stated matter-of-factly, then chattered on about how relieved he was that Simba would be getting shots and not die.

Tim's proclamation to anyone who would listen each morning was how many days were left until dog license day. On the morning of the twenty-second, Tim woke us at 6:00 with the surprise announcement: "This is the day my dog gets his shot!"

The clinic was not open until 7:00 that evening. I was sure

that Tim's state of anticipation would wear him out before the day was over.

He hardly ate his supper and was raring to go long before it was time. But when we drove up to the enormous supermarket parking area, it was packed with cars, people, and dogs. A line four blocks long wove in and out. I knew it would be at least nine o'clock before we ever reached the booth.

"Why don't we go to the Humane Society tomorrow and get Simba's shot, and then we can go to city hall and get the license?" I suggested.

"No! No!" Tim persisted.

"But you'll have to wait at least *two hours*!"

"I don't care. I'll wait." Tim opened the car door and started for the line. Simba was straining at his leash. The sight of all the other dogs excited him, and he dragged Tim toward the line.

"I need my jacket. Why don't you go get a book to read?" Tim called to me.

When I brought Tim his jacket, he was patiently waiting. And stand we did. I was grateful that I'd recovered from my knee injury because we stood and walked and walked and stood. The dogs sniffed, barked, and growled at each other. To mark the now five-block line of people and dogs, orange-shaped cones were set out and were dutifully christened by the dogs.

It was almost 9:00 when we finally reached the stand where the shots were being given. Simba instinctively knew that he wanted no part of whatever was coming. Tim half carried, half dragged him up the stairs to the platform. When Tim put Simba down, he lay with his paws flat in front of him. Simba refused to budge, and Tim had to pull him by his collar. Simba skidded across the floor.

The veterinarian helped Tim lift Simba onto the table. Tim put both hands on Simba to help hold him down and turned his own head the other way. He couldn't bear the sight of his dog getting a shot. The vet winked at me and quipped to Tim, "We have shots on special. Would you like one?"

"No way! No way!" Tim replied emphatically.

Simba followed willingly as we entered the dog license line. "I sure hope they give us the metal tag tonight," Tim sighed.

When we arrived home it was just past nine. Right away Tim got the pliers, pried open the wire holder on the dog tag, and put it on Simba's collar. All the time he talked to Simba, "Now we don't have to worry anymore. If the dogcatcher gets you, we can get you back." Tim hugged Simba tightly and then let him outside.

One Thursday afternoon in early February Tim came prancing into the house, pulled two dimes out of his pocket, and plopped them on the table.

"Where'd the dimes come from? Haven't you been buying milk?" I questioned.

"Two kids at school bought my chocolate chip cookies."

"The mothers would be unhappy if they knew their children were buying cookies with milk money."

"Oh, no." Tim's eyes widened. "It's their ice-cream money."

"Are you sure?"

"Yaaah! I'm sure." He turned and went to his room and brought out five dimes. "See, I've made fifty cents!"

"Tim, I think you better stop selling your cookies. I don't think the mothers of those kids or the school would like it."

"But the kids really like your cookies, Mom. I trade mine for store-bought Twinkies and cupcakes," Kevin chimed in.

"You what? I don't bake cookies for you guys to sell and trade away. I'm not going to bake anymore, if you keep doing this."

"But, Mom!" the boys chorused.

Tim giggled and put his arms around me. "The kids love your cookies."

"And they don't like the store kind. You never buy the store stuff, and we can get all the cookies we want at home," Kevin interjected with his so-called selling point.

Before I could protest anymore, Tim had let Simba in. He flew past Kevin and me. A yelping-yelling Tim-Simba commotion broke out in the living room. I settled them down, then went to finish cleaning our bedroom.

A couple of hours later when I went to prepare dinner, I couldn't find the steak that had been thawing on the counter. I looked all over, behind the coffeepot, under clutter, and inside the refrigerator, thinking the boys might have put it in there. But no steak!

In the middle of my search I stopped, muttering to myself, "Now, I'm sure I put a round steak out to thaw. It was right here." Putting my hand on the counter, I stepped forward and my foot landed on a small hard object. It was a small round white bone, with only a small piece of pink still attached.

"THE DOG! He ate the steak!"

Simba had long since been banned to the backyard. The boys were down the street playing. I was talking to nobody. I stuck my head out the open window and yelled at the dog, "You bad dog! You ate our supper!"

Later, Tim came in to check on supper, a habit he'd developed. "What are we having for supper?"

"You'll find out when we sit down." I didn't want to hear his usual complaints.

Tim reached for the oven door, pulled it open, and peered inside. "Yukkk! Meat loaf! I thought we were having steak. You know I hate meat loaf."

"Well, your dog got ahold of the steak and ate it up."

"He did? You're kidding!"

"No, I'm not."

"Really, you mean it?"

"Honest."

Tim laughed, then frowned. "I still hate meat loaf. I don't want to eat."

It really wouldn't have mattered what we were having for

dinner. Tim's food tastes are completely unpredictable. His appetite is hearty, but it seems that what one day is a favorite food will become the object of intense dislike the next.

When we sat down at the table, Tim tipped his chair back. "I'm not going to eat that crappy meat loaf! Nothing's good to eat," he snarled.

"If you don't eat now, you can't have anything to eat after supper," Ron ordered. "Now put your chair down and eat!"

I reached across the table and started spooning food up for Tim. I wanted to make sure he got some of everything, because he wouldn't take it himself. And when he did help himself, he spilled food all over.

"What are you doing, providing butler service for Tim?" Kevin quipped. "You wouldn't do that for me."

"I've been saying that for a long time. Tim needs to do it for himself. He can dish up his own food," Ron put in.

"You're right," I agreed.

For too long our once pleasurable fun and fellowship mealtimes had been ruined with Dad-Mom-Tim verbal battles over what Tim didn't like and wasn't going to eat.

Eating was frustrating for Tim because his coordination was poor. He tore his bread when he spread butter on it, knocked things over, and spilled his food. He would pick up a piece of food, put it on the fork or spoon, drop it on the way to his mouth, then eat it with his fingers anyway. Because of his pick-it-up-and-spill-it eating method, the table, chair, and floor around him looked like a disaster area.

Yet we knew the only way he'd ever learn was to do things for himself. I wondered if half of Tim's hassling resulted from his oppositional food tastes and his easily irritated digestive system.

How we came upon the solution, I don't know. I think it was out of desperation. That evening we took Tim's tactics, turned them around, and mocked the food. Ron is especially good at subtle and sometimes silly teasing. (Our humor, however, never includes ridicule of a person; we direct it to the problem.)

Ron's eyes twinkled. "This food is awful. It's the worst meat loaf I've ever tasted."

Kevin joined in. "Yukkk! This is terrible."

"Uggh!" I wrinkled my nose.

And we all broke out laughing. We continued to agree with Tim's "the-food-is-awful" bit, and slowly, over the next weeks and months, he complained less often.

By Sunday, February 17, Tim had earned enough points marking words down from the pastor's sermon to go to the ice-cream parlor. Ron had to pick Kevin up from snow camp in the evening, so I agreed to take Tim for ice cream.

The ice-cream parlor tingled with bright lights, bells, and booming drums. The waiters and waitresses were dressed in gay nineties costumes, and the hubbub of happy noises gave us a carnival feeling.

Instead of just ordering a small ice-cream sundae, Tim wanted what was called a pig's trough. It had about three times as much ice cream as a regular sundae.

"Tim, you know that when you eat too much sugar it sets you off and you can't control yourself."

"Please, Mom?" Tim begged. "I'll control myself. I worked hard and have my heart set on a pig's trough."

"All right," I relented. "But you may have a difficult time at school tomorrow. You'll have to promise to try extra hard to control yourself."

"I will, Mom. Please?" he pleaded.

When Tim was finished gobbling down his pig's trough, the waitress appeared and asked Tim to stand up. To gain everyone's attention she held her hand above Tim and shouted, "This young man has earned the prize of pig and has won a ribbon for his nose!" She stuck a green ribbon imprinted with "I made a pig of myself" on his nose. "At the count of three on the big bass drum, everyone yell, 'Oink—oink—suey—suey,' in recognition of this feat."

Tim beamed as the entire parlor packed with people yelled, "Oink—oink—suey—suey."

The next day Mrs. Davis called after school. Her voice was shaking. "Mrs. Cragg, can you come to school right away? Tim was doing his spelling assignment during reading class, and I've kept him after school to complete it, but he has steadfastly refused to do it. He says I can't make him and thinks you won't come to school."

"I'll be right there," I stated. When I arrived at school, Tim was sitting in the office.

Tim was angry and sneered when Mrs. Davis told me, "Tim is belligerent and talks back when I try to get him to do his work."

"I'm not going to do the work! I don't have to," he challenged sarcastically.

"Yes, you do!" I took Tim by the arm and Mrs. Davis and I walked him to the reading room. We sat in small chairs on either side of Tim.

"I'm not going to do any work." He crossed his arms and tipped his chair back.

"If we have to sit here until seven or eight tonight, we will wait until you're done."

A garble of unintelligible complaints spewed from Tim.

"Tim, we can't understand what you are saying."

"I didn't want . . . " a jumble of words tumbled forth again.

"Tim, say it slowly."

"Never mind. Just forget it!" He crossed his arms.

"Tim, we want to know."

"You never understand what I say."

"I'm sorry. But you need to calm down. Explain slowly." (The inability to be understood has always been frustrating for Tim. Even when he's not angry he has a difficult time expressing himself clearly.)

"I didn't want to do the work because I wouldn't have any

playtime," he stumbled. He flipped his hand toward Mrs. Davis. "She talked so fast I didn't understand the directions."

"If you understood the top part then you should have understood the bottom. They were the same. I've been telling you that if you can't get your work done you should take it home. I can't let you do spelling during reading class."

"Dad helped you with your math the other night," I reminded Tim. "You know we'll help you. Why haven't you brought your work home?"

"But I want to play after school."

Both Mrs. Davis and I started to reason with Tim and I knew we were trapped on that spiraling, whirling challenge-explain-argue-go-round. "This is enough! We're not going to discuss it anymore. You have to do your work."

"Tim, your reading folder is in the closet," Mrs. Davis interjected.

Tim rose and swiped his hand across a table, spilling a stack of reading cards all over the floor.

I stood. "Tim, pick them up. Put them on the table the way they were."

Tim scowled, but picked the cards up. He shoved them every which way, then started to dump them on the table.

He strode over to the closet and deliberately yanked on the locked part where the children kept their jackets and lunch pails.

His teacher was standing behind us. "Tim, you know that your folder is not in there."

Tim jerked open the door to the left and pulled the box of folders out. He fussed, fumed, and pawed over the folders, not really looking for his own. When he couldn't find it, he finally settled down and went through each one. "It's not here!"

Mrs. Davis took the box out of Tim's hand and found that it had accidentally been clipped to another folder. When she unclipped it and handed it to Tim, the folder fell on the floor and papers spilled all over.

Tim reached down to pick them up. He jerked one drawing

back and forth. "See this pig I drew. It's my teacher!"

My insides sank. I was sick. His remark stunned me and I was speechless.

When he sat at the table, Tim announced, "My teacher will have to stay here while I do my work. She can't leave!"

"I have other important things to do," Mrs. Davis wisely stated, and left the room. She was not going to let Tim manipulate her with his threat.

As soon as she was gone, Tim laid his arms on the table and buried his head. Surging sobs welled up. His body shook. "You shouldn't have let me eat that ice cream," he sobbed, pouring his feelings out for a long time. Finally he quieted down enough to do his work. But he was so emotionally distraught by now that his writing was erratic and almost illegible.

When he finished we took his work to Mrs. Davis and she excused him to go home. "Tim started the first thing this morning. He's been working up to it all day. He seemed full of electricity. It was really strange." (Mrs. Davis had never witnessed an electrical outburst.)

"We let him stay up too late last night and let him have too much ice cream," I explained. "This was a serious mistake. It seems likc every time he eats too many sweets he can't control himself as well. I'm really sorry," I apologized. "Thank you so much. We really appreciate everything you've done."

We talked some more about the pressures on Tim and the work he was unable to do. Then she thanked me for coming and giving my support. I was heartsick as we left for home. I knew Tim really loved Mrs. Davis, but it grieved me that he had treated her the way he did.

It took this one dramatic, tragic episode to bring home to us that too much sugar really did trigger tantrums in Tim. After that day Tim was convinced that he could not drink cola or orange juice, or eat excessive amounts of sweets, and donuts in particular.

We'd continued to pray that our health insurance would pay

for Tim's therapy and that I would be able to have the hysterectomy soon. Within a few days each of these prayers was answered.

My gynecologist scheduled me for surgery the Tuesday after Easter. Then a check arrived in the mail to cover the cost of therapy. We were joyous! But our joys seemed to be seasoned with disappointments. Regretfully, we would never be able to resume therapy again because of financial limitations and my surgery. Bill's insights had helped us find new perspectives, and the sessions benefited us as much or more than Tim. I appreciated Bill's compassion and the sensitive way he guided us.

In our last session Bill said, "I talked with Mrs. Johnson about Tim attending a learning disability class part of the day. She said there are no openings and doubts if there will be for the rest of the year. I have some educational materials that you can order to help Tim in his problem areas."

We leafed through the literature, but I had to answer futilely, "I honestly can't do it right now. I'm threadbare emotionally. Pain has broken what little strength I have. My patience is thin. I'm afraid there's nothing more of me to give," I agonized. "Ron's days are long because he covers a large section of California. Sometimes he has to travel away from home. His evenings are tied up in paperwork and reports.

"After school is hard on Tim because he needs time to run off steam. He already resents therapy cutting into his playtime. Doing small amounts of homework is bad enough. He needs more free time than most children.

"You know, Bill," I softly spoke, "love is not enough. Who we are—will be—or ever want to be is not enough. We can be ourselves with Kevin. We can get mad or sad or sick, and he adjusts. Yet our every reaction, every word with Tim, has to be measured, weighed, and balanced. We can't relax. Are we doing this right? Or are we wrong? We should do this. Or we should do that. Sometimes I would just like to be *me*," I sighed.

18

Resurrection and Renewal

Tim and David decided to put up the tent and sleep outside. We'd been having summer weather in March. At 6:30 the next morning Ron was leaving for a men's prayer breakfast. Tim and David didn't hear Ron as he stood listening by their tent for a few minutes before leaving. The boys were having morning devotions by reading their Bible aloud together.

After breakfast, and all on his own, Tim decided that this was the day to trim the hedge. He asked if David and he could earn some money. They started their trimming attack at nine. Tim was so earnest that he paused briefly for lunch and kept right on clipping until six o'clock that evening. David, tiring, threw sticks for Simba, then went home after lunch because Tim wouldn't both work and play.

Our neighbor, Mr. Upton, came out in the afternoon to check on the hedge cutting and complained that the hedge was too low. I don't think he appreciated its rolling hills appearance. Even though the hedge is actually on his property line, Tim is the only one who has kept it clipped over the past four years.

When Tim came dragging into the house it was almost dark. I expected him to collapse from exhaustion. I wrapped both my arms all the way around him, gave him a hug, and nestled my nose in his ear, "You know something—"

"I love you," Tim giggled quietly.

"You did an excellent job on the hedge. I'm really proud of you," I praised.

"Yes, son, you really worked hard. Thanks!" Ron patted Tim on the shoulders.

This whispered You-know-something-I-love-you exchange delights Kevin and Tim. I've done this with them since they were toddlers. Praise is one of the most wholesome ingredients of love. It nourishes the acceptable.

The neighborhood gang, John, Johnny, Brian, Lawrence, and Sid showed up at 8:00 with the unison request, "Can we put up the tents in your yard and sleep out tonight?"

Tim perked up, and that well of energy that bubbles forth from him overflowed. "Let me sleep out again? *Honest*, I'm not too tired. Please, Mom, please! Can we?"

I looked to Ron to seek his decision. "It's all right with me. But you boys will have to quiet down early. Tomorrow is church."

The boys agreed to attend church with us and dropped their Sunday clothes on our cedar chest and couch. Snacks, tents, tools, tarps, blankets, pillows, flashlights, ropes, stakes, sleeping bags, comic books, shoes, socks, marbles, rocks, treasures, and boys were scrambled, scattered, and spread all over our front porch and yard.

The boys strung ropes from the tree, pounded in the stakes, pitched two backpack tents, and attached one makeshift blanket affair to the house. I couldn't figure out how they were able to separate and sort everything out, but they managed.

Then the hassling and haggling started.

"I wanna sleep here."

"No! I do."

"I don't care."

"Well, Johnny and I are sleeping in this tent."

"We are!"

"No, you're not."

"You can sleep there. We'll sleep here."

"But I don't like the blanket tent."

"Tough!"

This set off a light skirmish. They finally agreed on who belonged where, popped several bowls of popcorn, drank punch and water to wash it down, and then supposedly settled in for the night.

"Ouch! Ouch! Ouch!" Six-foot, two-inch John danced out of the tent in his skivvies. Ant armies had attacked.

Swatting boys jumped and jiggled around the yard trying to rid themselves of the pesky enemy. Their encampment was directly over an anthill.

Stakes were torn up, tents and tarps, blankets and bags were shaken out. It was 10:30 when the tents were finally erected again. But the blankets kept collapsing. The tents sagged. The ants' radar equipment searched the boys out and the biting siege began again.

Our promised early bedtime was pushing 11:00 P.M. One by one the boys straggled into the house and sacked out in their sleeping bags. We had wall to wall bodies in our small living room. Just get a group of guys together and their jokes and hee-hawing outdoes any gathering of giggling girls.

Ron and I couldn't help but laugh at some of their silly shenanigans, but if we were going to make it through the services without sleeping, they'd have to calm down. Tim was wide-awake, wound up, and wild. He pranced and hopscotched over all the boys, bugging and teasing them. When we got him to calm down and into his sleeping bag, the hee-haws quieted to whispering snickers. And I think we finally fell asleep about midnight.

The next morning I stepped gingerly over disheveled bags filled with dozing, drowsy, stretching, yawning, rumple-haired boys, trying to make my way to the kitchen.

"Fix us some pancakes, Mom?" Kevin asked.

"Yeahhh!" agreed the gang.

One-hundred-and-seventy-pound, five-foot-four-inch Johnny incited a pancake-eating contest with, "I bet I can eat more pancakes than you can."

"No, you can't! I can."

"No, I can!"

"You can't either."

The volley of challenges bounced back and forth between the boys.

Because of Tim's restricted sugar intake, he didn't join the contest. The other boys gave out at four and five pancakes each. But tall John and Johnny kept going: five—ten—fifteen—twenty. John heaved a sigh and gave up; he was stuffed. Johnny won with a record of twenty-four pancakes. Altogether I think I served sixty-three pancakes that morning.

On March 26 Mrs. Feinberg, the district psychologist whom I had never met, surprised me with a phone call.

"I tested Tim. I'd like to know if you can come to school tomorrow at 1:00 to discuss the results."

"Ahh—fine. See you tomorrow." The phone clicked, and the buzzing left me with that hanging-in-the-air feeling. I didn't know they were testing Tim.

At school the next day I waited only a few minutes until a slender woman with brick-red hair, a splash of freckles, and snapping hazel eyes appeared. She was dressed in emerald green slacks, matching turtleneck, and checked shirt-jacket.

"Mrs. Cragg?"

"Yes." I stood.

"Mrs. Feinberg." She turned and motioned. "Let's go into the nurse's office."

We sat in child-size chairs. She opened Tim's folder, tipped her chair back, crossed her legs, and shot questions at me in rapid order. She was straightforward and used the let's-lay-it-all-on-the-table approach.

"He's got quite a folder here for not having any difficulties at school!" (All test results from the past had been forwarded by the district. Tim's folder was understandably thick.)

She started her questioning at Tim's birth and progressed to the present. How many times I'd answered all this before.

"I'm sorry I had to put Tim through these tests again," Mrs. Feinberg apologized. "He's been tested too much already. But it's the only way I can place him in the program."

Again, as before, I replied, "Yes, I know he's been tested too much."

Reliving the past and reviewing Tim's long history of testing and over-testing was not easy. Candidly and matter-of-factly I briefly explained why we wanted Tim in a learning disability class. To me his needs were obvious.

"Well," she countered, "Tim's reading scores are higher than his test last October with Dr. Walters. He's only a year behind in his reading ability, which disqualifies him for special reading. But his math scores show him to be two years behind. We can place him in a one-hour math program."

"But he's supposed to be in the fifth grade, not fourth," I protested. "According to these scores that would make him two years behind in reading, and three years in math."

"We're just considering where he is right now. Not where he should be."

"What about Tim's inability to understand or read directions?" I asked. "This seems to be where he needs the most help."

"He's come up in the area of understanding instructions. Every verbal direction I gave, he repeated aloud. That's all right. It's his way of compensating." (This was not an entirely accurate deduction. Tim did not and could not repeat instructions out loud in class as he read them. According to Mrs. Davis he could do very little of his work unless she went to his desk and explained everything. Then and only then could Tim proceed.)

"Why has it been so difficult to get Tim into this class before now?" I sighed.

"It's in the borderline, slow-learning category that we get the most complaints from parents, because funded programs are not available," Mrs. Feinberg explained.

"The state will provide money for the 2 percent in the higher intelligence brackets, the 2 percent with lower intelligence, then special areas such as hard of hearing or blind children. But Tim is not a slow learner; the IQ tests brought him above that this time."

"If Tim had disturbed the class more than he has, would they put him in an educationally handicapped class without our requesting it?"

Mrs. Feinberg didn't answer. I knew it didn't matter whether the child was a slow learner or a genius; if he were consistently uncontrollable he would be transferred to special classes or removed entirely. Public education is mandatory with the exception of the child who is disruptive; then the rule changes.

"Who's Tim's doctor?" she asked.

"Dr. Kenyon."

"Oh, yes. He's a good man. He knows what he's doing. What drug is Tim taking now?"

"Dilantin. Dr. Walters states that Tim has subclinical nonconvulsive epileptic syndrome. Along with the vitamins he takes, I feel the Dilantin has made a significant difference."

"Tim needs to learn to be responsible for his own actions," she advised. "He needs to suffer the consequences of poor choices and what he does wrong." Mrs. Feinberg then recommended a well-known book on the subject.

"Dr. Walters uses a reward type of system in which Tim earns points for the right kind of actions and self-control."

"I don't believe in that at all!" she retorted. "Children have to learn to become a responsible part of the family. No one should get a reward for behaving."

"I've had some difficulty with the reward system, because sometimes it works and sometimes it doesn't," I explained. "But I respect Dr. Walters' opinion; he's the first person who's made any sense. I feel he's clearly pinpointed Tim's difficulties."

Mrs. Feinberg pulled out some pamphlets which supported her particular point of view. "Tim's highly manipulative," she said.

"Yes, he is."

"That in itself indicates that Tim is not a slow learner. It shows he's able to think. A slow learner would not be able to do that."

She changed the topic of conversation again. "In two weeks there's going to be a four-hour hearing at the district office. There's plenty of room in the learning disability class here at this school. There'll be no problems whatsoever placing Tim in the program. You can come to the hearing if you like, but there will be no need of it, because my recommendation guarantees his placement." She concluded crisply, then stood and opened the door to the breezeway.

I started to walk away, but I hadn't thought to ask exactly when Tim would be placed in the math class. I just assumed September was the soonest available spot. That the possibility was immediate hadn't entered my mind. Something compelled me to turn back. "Oh, by the way, when will Tim be able to get into the class?"

"In the middle of April."

A stunned silence swept over me. It was obvious that Mrs. Feinberg was totally unaware of what we had been told in the past about long waiting lists, children with more severe problems needing help first, a class that was full, and that he wasn't far enough behind.

Mrs. Feinberg felt her observations were valid. But without exception, every psychologist, medical doctor, or other professional we've consulted has had a different opinion, perspective, diagnosis, and label! The vastly different methods of solving Tim's disabilities and the varied diagnoses have caused confusion.

As parents we've had to analyze the analyses. Who's right? Who's wrong? I'll always remember the first school psychologist who tested Tim when he was in the first grade. The psychologist told me that children with celiac disease often grow up to be recluses, plus a few other predictions that shattered my day.

We couldn't begin to share all the labels that have been tagged to Tim for fear they would have adverse affects on his future well-being. As time passes, the majority have proven to be groundless.

Clearly, Tim was hyperactive and had learning problems. The confusion rested in this multiple question: Did Tim also have epilepsy or a psychological disorder or was he just being manipulative? Dr. Walters' diagnosis of epilepsy proved to be correct.

When I informed Ron about the math class that would begin in April, he jubilantly announced, "Well, we have other good news. I'm getting a hundred dollar raise in the middle of April!"

Our financial situation had been on the skids for several months because of the spiraling cost of living and our mounting medical bills.

Easter Sunday was centered in the middle of April. The prayers that had been on our hearts for months and even years were to be answered simultaneously. My long-awaited surgery was scheduled for Tuesday after Easter. Tim was going to his class after the spring vacation, which was the first Monday after Easter, and Ron's raise would be coming the Friday before Easter.

My faith in God, whose plans are providential, had been tested and tried. I had begun to believe that, yes, God is there, but He allowed us to endure life's valleys without His intervention.

To some, this triangle of prayers which were to be answered at Easter time would seem coincidental, but nothing with God is by accident.

During spring, as the budding of new life awakened after its long winter hibernation, the hope of resurrection and renewal was coming to our family.

19

Role Reversal

It was a quiet summer. Kevin worked full time as a junior staff member at the Boys Club. Three weeks he was away on two backpacking trips.

Tim and I stayed home. I needed rest. My recuperation from surgery was slow, and pain persisted. Gradually a new kind of calm, self-control, self-direction, and motivation had taken hold on Tim's life.

Tim's summer-to-school transition was smooth, without any surging waves of hyperactivity and hostility. Tim, now eleven, would be entering fifth grade. His favorite teacher, Mrs. Davis, had retired to stay home with her infant son.

It wasn't until school had been in progress a couple of weeks that we were surprised by the unexpected—rotating classes and teachers. One of the reasons Tim had been transferred from the school he'd previously attended was because we did not feel he could adjust to changing classes. This program was to be a modified form, but I questioned it. Too many changes confuse Tim.

After a talk with Mrs. Johnson we agreed that Tim was possibly mature enough to cope. It would give him the opportunity to prepare for moving from class to class in junior high school, which was only two years away.

But Tim didn't adjust to the program, could not settle down or concentrate on his work. He complained that he was confused and came home with headaches. The team of teachers made a special effort to work with Tim; they understood his limitations, with the exception of one teacher. Mr. Fogg and Tim clashed constantly. Conferences and phone calls increased with frequency those first few weeks.

Mr. Fogg lost his temper. He pushed and shoved the children around. His nagging tirades earned him the title of Croaky the Frog among the children.

Mr. Fogg did attempt several methods to reestablish proper classroom environment and build a rapport with the children. Mrs. Johnson kept in constant touch with the situation and worked with Mr. Fogg. But the stage was set from the beginning, and the chaotic conditions in his class continued.

In late October, we had our first parent-teacher conference. In Tim's regular classes it was only a goal-setting conference. But the report that Mr. Lee, Tim's soft-spoken oriental special education teacher, filled out for the learning disability math class was perplexing. Almost everything was checked both "yes" and "no."

As I looked over the report my puzzled expression must have revealed my feelings. "Tim has a difficult time settling down," Mr. Lee explained. "Some days he sits down and does his work without any direction. Other times he wanders around, opens his work, then closes his book halfway through class, and puts it all away."

Mr. Lee turned to Tim. "What would happen when you grow up and go to work if one day you feel like working and the next day you don't?"

"I'd be fired," Tim shot back.

"Most children with learning problems are like this," Mr. Lee told me later. "They seem to master a subject completely, such as understanding the exchange value of money. Then later they completely forget what they learned. They have to start all over again and relearn it. Only it isn't as difficult as before, because it comes back quicker. I imagine Tim will always be this way, and he'll have to learn how to compensate and live with it."

Tuesday morning, November 5, Tim announced, "Guess what? I think I took two pills last night."

"What makes you think that?" I inquired.

"I'm so sleepy. And Jimmy Garcia, a friend of mine, said he sneaks two extra pills to keep from becoming so hypo at school. And he takes the same blue pills I used to."

I discussed the dangers of taking an extra pill with Tim. This was the first time we'd ever faced this problem. Tim desired so much to behave himself that he resorted to taking an extra pill.

I then clarified something that Tim hadn't realized. "Dr. Kenyon does not have you on a pill to stop you from being hyperactive. The pill you take is to stop the temper tantrums you used to have. Dr. Kenyon said he won't give you anything to control your 'hypos,' so you're going to have to help yourself and try harder."

Since that one episode we've had no more problems with him taking an extra pill. But one time a couple of months later, Tim forlornly remarked, "I sure wish you'd let me take two pills so I can control my hypos at school." It had been a painful struggle, and it hurt; and the hurt was indescribable.

On Friday, November 8, Tim barged into the house. Deep gasping breaths heaved his entire body, scarlet red flushed his face, and perspiration stood out like pearls on his forehead. He shook. His eyes were wide and horror-stricken.

"What's the matter?"

"That Mr. Frog chased me home. But I got away from him."

"What for?"

"I got in a fight with Frankie. Mr. Frog came after me in his *car*! He chased me in and out of some apartments, but I ran fast. His car screeched and whirled in the dust. He couldn't find me, and I got out of there!" Tim's hands flailed the air; he depicted the entire scene with his body.

"I think we better go right back to school and straighten this out!"

"No! No!"

"Yes, we'll have to." Tim was so keyed up I expected him to explode, but he only protested mildly.

I was torn between two opinions. On the one hand I was frightened that Mr. Fogg would pursue Tim in his car. Tim's wild description called up images of a cops-and-robbers chase. On the other hand, I needed to know what Tim had done and why Mr. Fogg had felt the need to chase him.

When we walked into the outer office, Frankie was sitting on the floor. Mr. Fogg and Mrs. Johnson were having a conference in her office. The door was wide open. When Mr. Fogg saw us, he rose, "I was just going to call you."

"I came to see what happened," I answered simply.

"Would you please be seated; I'll be with you in a few minutes," Mrs. Johnson said matter-of-factly as she shut her door.

Tim and Frankie bantered and bickered back and forth. A few boys from class peeked through the door. They interrupted Frankie in the middle of telling me how Tim had beat him up.

"You deserved it, Frankie," they taunted.

"Yeah, you bugged Tim all day long."

"You wouldn't leave him alone."

"No—no I didn't," Frankie protested.

"Yes—yes you did," they chorused.

"You had it coming to you."

"You threw pencils at Tim. Remember!"

"You called him names during football."

I stopped the argument, and the secretary chased the boys off. The truth was that this was not the first time Frankie and Tim had clashed. Frankie was as high-strung as Tim, and they lit each other into a roaring bonfire. It was an equal blame situation.

A ninety-minute conference followed. First Mrs. Johnson, Mr. Fogg, and both boys met. Then Mrs. Johnson, Mr. Fogg, and Tim talked things over. And finally all of us met, with the exception of Frankie.

The reason Mr. Fogg gave for chasing Tim in the car was that he saw Tim at the apartments across the street pounding Frankie. Why Mr. Fogg didn't just run across the street and stop the fight, I never found out.

Despite Mr. Fogg's dangerous reaction we resolved a great deal that day. Mrs. Johnson urged Tim to come see her any time he was upset and needed someone to talk with.

Even though the confrontations continued between Mr. Fogg and Tim, some remarkable changes were taking place in Tim at home. Almost every day after school he'd burst forth with, "Do you wanna hear what Mr. Frog did today? He locked Jim in a closet." Or, "He ripped a boy's shirt." And again, "He scratched a girl's arm."

In the past a constant negative exchange like this set Tim off into uncontrollable hyperactivity or rage, but now it didn't. He verbalized his hostility and then went out to play.

I tried to balance the situation and not feed Tim's antagonism against Mr. Fogg. When I could clearly see that Tim was in the wrong I pointed it out and reminded him that there would always be Mr. Foggs in the world to contend with, and that Tim would get along much better if he would not deliberately defy him.

What we didn't realize was that Tim had done a complete role reversal. At home his behavior and reactions were normal. At school he was the exact opposite. By December all of Tim's teachers were upset and ready to have him transferred to a full-day program for the educationally handicapped.

Oddly, Tim felt he was doing fine at school. He didn't think he was having any problems with his teachers. He liked them all, except Mr. Fogg.

Two weeks before Christmas Ron and I met with Mrs. Feinberg, the district psychologist, and Mrs. Johnson for another lengthy session. Edith, a friend from Oregon, happened to be visiting us. A special education teacher, she joined us in the conference.

What concerned Ron and me was Tim's reversal. Mrs. Feinberg looked upon it more positively than we did. She felt it was better that Tim didn't bottle everything up and blow off only at home, which he had done in the past.

Now the school was faced with the full impact of Tim's behavior. Mrs. Feinberg felt this would give the staff the opportunity to help Tim even himself out and handle all situations. She promised to observe Tim in class, talk to teachers, write out an evaluation, and set up a program for Tim after Christmas vacation.

After our school conference, Edith and I talked the rest of the afternoon, into the early morning hours, and all the next day.

In that two-day talking/sharing marathon, God helped me gain renewed perspectives. Edith urged me to stop being concerned about academics. It wasn't that we expected Tim to be an above-average student. Even though Tim lagged behind, his reading ability was excellent and he mastered math concepts and other subjects in his own time. Comprehending the initial directions was impossible for him. It was our hope that he could learn to decipher instructions prior to junior high and high school, where teachers are unable to give individualized attention.

Edith felt Tim had mastered enough of the basics. She was impressed with his abilities despite his handicaps. For many adults, academics is a small part of daily living work experience. Tim's ability to relate to people, get along, follow the orders of a boss without becoming angry, and endure the bumps and bruises of life without failing were equally important.

But as parents it had been hard for us to accept Tim's learning handicaps, because he's very sharp. We had hoped that with proper visual and auditory perception exercises and individualized teaching, Tim would have broken some of those barriers. It seemed an impossible dream, and we had to recognize that Tim would have to compensate rather than conquer.

Edith felt Ron and I had done a great deal towards building independent, basic living habits through Tim's yard work and his experiences earning money at the Taylors.

God's purposes are never singular, but multiplied; His timing is incredible. Edith had come for her son's graduation and a two-day visit with us. Her coming at that time was a divine appointment. Her intelligent perceptions and added insights to our school conference were invaluable. She had interpreted the educator's viewpoint to us in layman's terms.

Tim's paradoxical behavior, however, of coping normally in one place but losing complete control at another baffled and haunted us. Ron and I earnestly prayed for guidance. We desired above all else to know how to help Tim, yet we were mystified. There seemed to be no sugarcoated solutions.

During the months of October through December, Tim had made one rewarding accomplishment. He had been working at the Taylors two days after school and a half day on Saturday. Shirley had contracted with a local factory to collate packages of guitar strings in numerical order. He earned a dollar a gross and his goal was to buy a brand-new Schwinn Sting-Ray, dirt bicycle.

In November, he'd picked out the accessories on the bright red beauty and put a down payment on it. One week before Christmas, the day before we were to pick up the bike, Tim requested, "Mom, when you get my money out of the bank, will you get a fifty-dollar bill? I've never seen one before and I want to hold it in my hand."

Ron and I took him to the bike shop the next day, and Tim proudly placed ninety-one dollars in cash on the counter. He could hardly contain himself, he was so thrilled.

Tim had failed miserably these past months at school. All of us rejoiced in the confidence-building success of Tim earning and buying a new bicycle all by himself—representing over ninety-one hours of hard work.

Gently we clasped the hand of the Christmas holiday. The two-week break was exactly the breather Tim and his teachers needed.

20

Unlocked Doors

In the spring we met for our parent-teacher conference. Mrs. Morrow and Mr. Washington, one of the other team teachers, said Tim seemed to be coping better. Mrs. Morrow had been keeping Tim out of Mr. Fogg's class as much as possible and indicated that Mr. Fogg would no longer be teaching at the school.

Mr. Lee, Tim's math teacher, was equally confident in Tim's improvement. Tim had progressed from his two-year deficiency in math. He had reached his own age and grade level in one year's time.

Mr. Fogg was replaced by another teacher the following week. With his absence and the teacher's confidence in Tim's improvement, I relaxed. Maybe now we would see some bright streams of hope.

One month later, a dark shade shut out the rays of light. When Mrs. Johnson phoned, her voice was quivering. "Tim has not been doing any better. The teachers have had about all they can stand. Maybe it would be best to send Tim back to the school he originally attended. I thought I'd transfer him tomorrow!"

I was stunned! Since Mr. Fogg's departure, Tim had been calm and relaxed at home. He was still giving us no indication at all that anything was seriously wrong at school. Everything he expressed was positive, and so we thought all was well.

"A change this late in the year would only be detrimental," I protested. But because Tim was attending his present school on an inner-district transfer, I knew the choice was not ours. It was entirely up to Mrs. Johnson whether or not to accept a student.

"We could try him on a minimum day," she suggested. "Instead of returning home at 3:00, he could go home at 12:15. We can see if he does better on a shorter day. He cooperates in the morning, but by afternoon he's totally out of control. Why don't you check with Dr. Kenyon?" she suggested. "Perhaps Tim needs his medication changed."

"Could you give me some specifics to tell the doctor?" I asked. "We'll also try to check with Dr. Walters."

The next morning Mrs. Johnson filled me in on Tim's problems. "When Tim has to make choices regarding interest centers, he sits in a lotus position with his feet on his desk, sprawls on the floor, or crawls under a table. It happens especially when he's doing committee work with other children.

"He needs to get his hair cut," Mrs. Johnson continued. "He pulls it in front of his face and hides. He doesn't acknowledge that he is listening, and he is unresponsive to the teachers. On the playground he's still acting like one of the Three Stooges. Another problem is that Tim has been twenty minutes to half an hour late to school every day for a couple of months," she concluded.

Apparently Tim had been dawdling all three blocks to school, and we were totally unaware of his tardiness. This was the first time it had been mentioned.

That evening when Ron and I discussed the situation with Tim, I asked, "Why didn't you let us know that you were having a hard time?"

"Because you'd *do* something about it, like you are now,"

he replied hopelessly.

Tim was compensating any way he could so we wouldn't "do something" about him. In order to live peacefully without any more hassling, and just survive, he'd suppressed everything.

We were again faced with unsolvable questions and the complexities of seeking medical and professional help. We could not ignore the seriousness of Tim's needs, and yet the constant probing was and is devastating. We prayed for a key to unlock the doors that closeted Tim.

When I called Dr. Kenyon's office I was informed that he was recuperating from surgery and it would be two months before he would return to his practice. Dr. Walters was also booked solid for a week and a half.

A nurse recommended Dr. Messenger to us, indicating that he specialized in preventive medicine. Fortunately, we were able to see him the following Wednesday.

When we met Dr. Messenger I knew right away that he was a man of gentle compassion, yet strong. During our initial conversation I learned that he knew Christ in an intimate way.

Dr. Messenger took a preliminary history and set up a battery of blood tests, one of which was to check Tim's blood sugar level. The following week his nurse took a sample of Tim's hair, which would be used to test for mineral imbalances. We were asked to keep a detailed account of all the foods Tim ate in a week.

The results of the blood tests showed no abnormalities, and Tim's sugar level was normal. Dr. Messenger prescribed vitamins and kept Tim on the Dilantin.

Even though the dosage of vitamins was increased gradually over a period of time, they upset Tim's digestion and caused stomach cramps. He became fidgety, high-strung, and hyperactive. He has always been nocturnal, but trying to get him into bed and settled at a decent hour became increasingly difficult.

Tim's crises continued through the close of school. Mrs.

Johnson formally requested that Tim be transferred and placed in full-day special education. We were relieved and felt a small class would be more suitable for Tim.

The district hearing was scheduled for the second week after school was out. Mrs. Feinberg informed us that we would be invited to come, but that it was unnecessary. The sessions were lengthy, she had no idea when Tim's case would be presented, and her recommendation guaranteed his placement. We didn't attend the meeting and confidently assumed he'd be accepted.

When I checked to see where Tim would be attending school I was told that he had been placed on a waiting list. There was no assurance that he would get into a class and no information regarding where he would attend school.

It's never been easy for us to express the anger or sense of betrayal we feel at times like this. There are many aspects that must be considered, not only our accountability but that of others.

Throughout the year we'd sometimes had weekly encounters with school personnel in our attempts as parents to solve Tim's problems at school. While Tim's exposure to Mr. Fogg's incompetency and violence had seriously contributed to Tim's deterioration, it was we who were held accountable for his behavior. We were the ones who were requested to seek professional help for him. Only later did we learn that even some of the stronger, more self-assured children had been crushed by Mr. Fogg's classroom, and that he had resigned under the threat of a lawsuit.

Additionally, we were informed that state aid would not be granted for private special education and we had found it financially impossible to pay the high tuition rates of private specialized schooling.

For several months Karen, my phone prayer partner, had the increasing confidence that some of the exact causes of Tim's problems would be clearly pinpointed. Earnestly we prayed daily, not only for the bleak school situation but that

God would reveal specific insights to Ron and me.

Repeatedly, I tried to rest in God's sovereignty. Too often I'd find myself dwelling on the circumstances, disposing of faith and confidence, and borrowing back doubt and despair.

In July I employed Tim, Kevin, and several of their friends to help us paint. It had been at least five years since we had painted, and we intended to do most of the inside of the house. The gang agreed to work every morning if I'd take them to the beach in the afternoons.

Even though Tim was earning money, he flitted in and out and acted silly. This was unusual because he is ordinarily responsible at jobs that require similar type labor. He irritated all of us. By the third morning he was electric. It was only 9:00.

"Huh. Huh! You wanna fight?" He danced around and waved a foam bat in our faces.

We tried to ignore him, but his agitated activity accelerated.

"Stop it, Tim. We've had enough. Get dressed and eat," I ordered angrily.

That was the match that lit the rage. To prevent Tim from attacking, Kevin grabbed his arms and held on to him. I stood in front to prevent Tim from injuring Kevin. Tim flailed and screamed. He was so strong and struggled so hard that he pulled us into the kitchen.

After about fifteen minutes Tim slumped forward. We thought it was over, but Tim was still irritated. He ran to his room, put on his pants, dashed out in his bare feet, mounted his bike, and pedaled around in a daze.

Two weeks later we were in Dr. Messenger's office for a consultation. Kevin happened to be with us. Dr. Messenger talked with Tim first, then asked me how I felt everything was going.

"Summer's a more relaxed time and he's been doing fine.

He did have a tantrum, though, his first in over a year."

"Yeah, while we were painting," Kevin remarked softly to himself.

"I honestly don't know what could have caused it. We've watched his diet. Nothing upsetting has—"

"While you were painting," Dr. Messenger interjected. "He's allergic to the paint. It's a petrochemical."

"But it was water-base latex."

"It was the paint," Dr. Messenger repeated. "Many people are allergic to petrochemicals. I have some women patients who are allergic to natural gas and must cook only with electric stoves." He told me about a disturbed woman who went into a psychotic spell whenever she smelled a felt-tip pen.

I was skeptical. I couldn't imagine that something like water-base paint or petrochemicals could precipitate a rage. I left Dr. Messenger's office with reservations.

Ron's business schedule had been unusually pressing. The only time we could take our vacation was the first week of school. Kevin was disappointed; it was his first year of high school and he didn't want to miss it.

For Tim, however, we felt it would be best. Opening week is always hectic until everyone settles into a routine. Hopefully everything would be calm following our vacation and Tim would have a better start. We left the week before school opened and the district still had Tim on a waiting list. He was scheduled to return to the same school.

Throughout our trip we discussed specific ways Tim could handle his school situation. He genuinely determined to work at self-control. He was looking forward to school and hoped he'd have one of his favorite teachers.

We returned late Saturday afternoon. A letter from the district awaited us. Tim had been placed in a special education class in a school five blocks away. To add to our shock, his teacher's name was Mr. Fogg.

Tim was distraught and wept openly. He swore he wasn't

going. Although Fogg is such an unusual name we couldn't believe it would be the same person. As it turned out, this was a different Mr. Fogg, but it was still another traumatic and unexpected adjustment. It was evident that our decision to keep Tim out of school had been a wise one. He would have been transferred in the middle of his first week.

Tim's new Mr. Fogg was an easygoing, soft-spoken, gentle person. He was perfectly suited to teach special children with educational and behavioral difficulties. Each desk in his room was partitioned to lessen the distractions. Each child was encouraged to decorate his own titled "office." There were only twelve children and their education was structured to meet individual needs. Tim adjusted quickly and made new friends.

With Dr. Messenger's guidance, we traced the times Tim became electrical and hyperactive. We checked to see exactly what happened prior to an incident, whether it was singular, isolated, or if it happened repeatedly. We soon found that not eating was as disturbing as eating the wrong foods.

Saturdays, if Tim waited until almost noon to eat and take his medication, he would spiral. One day he lost his lunch and waited to come home and eat. He was highly overactive. We noted that if his meals were delayed he reacted the same way.

In December I bought a different type of water-base latex paint and painted the kitchen. Exactly three days later at 8:30 A.M. Mr. Fogg phoned and requested that I come after Tim. Tim had suddenly become angry and had thrown a stapler which had struck another boy. Mr. Fogg had had to carry him bodily out of the room. Although I had been skeptical before, I was now convinced that paint in particular induced a tantrum in Tim. We'd have to move him out for a week if we were to finish our half-painted kitchen.

We also found that excessively hot, smoggy days affected Tim. After several such days, Tim arrived home disoriented. His speech was slurred and he was unable to complete his sentences.

Carbon monoxide fumes and other air pollutants were also

included in this battery of irritants. Tim had been filling his minibike with gasoline. It wasn't muffled and the fumes were strong.

One evening he flopped on the bed. "I was at Brian's and I had to get home and lie down. My head has a floaty feeling. I could tell I was having a seizure, but I couldn't stop it. I can't feel things when I touch them. I can't think and I go blank." This lasted about fifteen minutes and then he seemed all right again.

Another time early in the summer Tim had the same experience after he'd been riding his minibike for a long time.

In March, Karen remarked, "We need to pray for Tim. This is his rough time of the year." That one statement triggered a flood of realizations.

We were in an area that is densely populated with a wide variety of trees, flowers, weeds, orchards, and grassy fields. Everything was freshly blooming. It was allergy season. Over the years, Tim had suffered his most critical crises during spring and fall. His behavior had reached such extremes during March that *all three EEGs had been scheduled in April*. Dr. Messenger concurred that pollen is an irritant and rejoiced that we had detected yet another environmental allergy.

We did not discover easy answers or simple cures. During our counseling sessions with Dr. Messenger he tried to help Tim realize that he will have to cope with these complexities for the rest of his life.

Tim faced it seriously. "What will I do when I grow up and need to paint my house?" was only one of a dozen questions he asked us.

Diet, vitamins, and protein supplements proved to be another paradoxical problem. Dr. Messenger doesn't view vitamin therapy as "the cure." We had hoped, however, that it would make a substantial change, as it has in some children. Tim takes vitamins, but massive doses were not effective.

Brewer's yeast, which is the basis of many B-complex vitamins, whole grains, and powdered high protein supplements in the minutest amounts cause Tim severe stomach cramps and sometimes result in diarrhea. At first I thought Tim was being oppositional and so I disguised protein powders or yeast in an eggnog drink. Only a few sips made him sick. His system immediately knew the difference between eggnog that had only a quarter of a teaspoon of powder and one that had none.

Although the elimination of foods which contain additives and colorings has been helpful in some children, we have not been able to embrace such a diet totally. This is because the list of foods that Tim cannot eat due to sugar content is endless, and the list of nutritionally vital foods that he cannot tolerate is equally long.

Our meals and snacks consist mainly of fresh meats, vegetables, fruits, nuts, and cheeses. We do not eat commercially prepared, packaged, frozen meals or casseroles. We avoid sugar-flavored fruit drinks, colas, and orange juice almost entirely. When we faithfully maintain this diet and don't become too lax, it makes a difference.

This past year has been a year of discovery. Tim has suffered few disruptive moments, and his improvement has been considerable. The sheltered structure of a small classroom has been ideal.

In retrospect, the vision of the past was clear and the view of our present moments dim. One time the road to regression was the path we trod, but we have found the path of progress.

We know that the years ahead are crucial years, and we are doing our utmost to prepare Tim to be responsible for himself. Just as a diabetic must live as normally as possible within his limitations, so must Tim monitor his life within his limitations. I sense within him a courageous desire to meet this task.

A year ago I found Tim's last and only teddy bear, long since discarded. It was on my sewing desk with a pile of other toys he no longer wanted. Its beige body was battered and bruised. The fur was skinned off in patches. Teddy's foot was bandaged, and Simba's teeth marks had punctured the tape.

The bear's backside had a bald spot, but his tail was intact.

His underarm was torn, and bits of old yellow foam trickled out. His tummy was empty, starved from not enough foam to fill it. His glass orange eyes appealed to me, and I thought to myself, "If only you could speak, there would be so many tales you could tell."

I picked the bear up and gently held it in my arms, and looked into its face. *We welcomed you into our home at Christmastime when Tim was not yet two and Kevin wasn't even four. You weren't alone; you came with three bear brothers, who've long since left home.*

Sometimes you were ignored.

Sometimes cradled.

Sometimes forgotten.

You've soothed tears away, weathered tantrums and dog bites.

And the adventures you've had? Water battles in mudholes. Dump truck and red wagon rides. Trips to the tree fort and a few free flights to the rooftop. Diagnoses and shots from Dr. Tim; you were an excellent patient.

Excursions away from home weren't happy unless you were along. And the places you've lived! Under the bed, in a closet, out in the morning dew, perched on a limb, in an old boat, but mostly snuggled safely next to a pillow—you've seen them all.

Sometimes lost.

Always found.

Always loved. You were his favorite.

Slowly I walked through the kitchen to the garage. "Tim, do you want your teddy bear?"

"No," he answered softly.

"Do you want me to put him in the Goodwill bag?"

Tim shook his head.

"What do you want me to do with your bear?"

Tim paused and thought momentarily. "Mom, would you save my teddy bear in the hope chest for a souvenir?"

Carefully I laid Tim's last teddy bear to rest, nestled among his baby blankets, infant outfits, pictures, and booties. Buried. Never to be forgotten; always to be a treasured keepsake.

Epilogue

Celebrations usually fade in my memory, blending into a potpourri of fragrant remembrances. Two festive observances will always remain as distinct memories for me. This past June Ron and I celebrated our silver anniversary and Tim graduated from high school. These occasions closed one season in our lives and marked the beginning of a new one.

At graduation we happened to sit next to a family whose son, Eric, had attended the same special education class with Tim for two years in junior high. Their teacher had prepared them for regular classes in high school. As we reminisced with Eric's parents, we all expressed our gratitude because—despite our mutual concerns and the difficulties we had experienced in the past—our sons were graduating.

During the ceremonies the graduates in their green or gold caps and gowns laughed and joked, wept and hugged one another, knowing they would never be together this way again. Many, like Tim, felt the regrets of leaving behind the freedom of youth for the responsibilities of adulthood.

We watched with affection as Tim said his good-byes to his friends while they grouped arm-in-arm for dozens of clicking cameras. In the silver anniversary edition of the yearbook under the heading *The Favorites of the Stars* . . . Tim had been listed among the "Class Clowns." He didn't disappoint his classmates now; he entertained them with his humorous banter and exaggerated poses, his cap and gown comically askew.

Earlier that week our sons and my parents had surprised us with a silver anniversary celebration. For three months they and Kevin's girlfriend, Kathy, had planned the event. When we walked into the reception room, Kathy handed me a bouquet and I found myself walking down the aisle on the arm of my father. Ron and I renewed our vows before Dick Grauer, our childhood friend and former pastor.

Ron and I were genuinely surprised and spent most of our celebration in euphoric shock as we greeted some forty friends and family members who had gathered to bring us joy. Kevin and Kathy added to our elation by announcing their engagement.

Kevin, now 21, produced a multi-media slide presentation. With a recording of Kenny Rogers singing "Through the Years," Kevin showed slides of our wedding and of our family during the boys' growing up years. The song seemed to capture the essence of our life together—of not remembering when we loved anyone else (Ron was 21 and I was 18 when we married). Through the years we held on to God's strength and to each other when everything went wrong. We struggled to work things out and we were grateful we had.

Looking back over these years, Ron and I were thankful God chose us to be Tim's special parents. But I wondered what Tim felt about his life. One afternoon I asked Tim, now 19, if he would share his thoughts about his high school years and his life now. (Today Tim works nights as a school custodian and plans to take automotive classes in college to become a diesel or Volkswagen specialist.)

While we talked, Tim stretched his lanky, 5'11″ muscular frame across his bed. His two walls of bookshelves were filled with records, Bibles, prom photos, yearbooks, motor repair manuals, and a red and gold crepe paper crown and trophy (his class voted Tim prom king his senior year). His red bubble gum machine, wearing Tim's blue felt hat, looked like a faceless midget guarding the door. Old-fashioned newsprint wallpaper covered the walls. His calendar hung open over his redwood desk and the verse beneath October 3 read: "Being confident of this very thing, that he which hath begun a good work in you will perform it until the day of Jesus Christ. Philippians 1:6."

As Tim talked about the previous summer, his sometimes serious, sometimes mischievous blue eyes accented his ruddy complexion. David, Brian, and he had gone with a Teen Missions evangelism team to England, and he was expressing how it affected his senior year in high school.

"While I was in England, I found out what I needed was a deeper commitment and relationship to the Lord. During this time I was able to share about my life with other people, their need of becoming Christians, and what God was all about. I realized I not only needed to be an effective witness on the mission field, but also at home and in school.

"At the beginning of my senior year, I met and became close to some neat Christians. We had lunchtime Bible studies, and many people at school made a commitment through our campus ministry. My last year of high school was probably one of my best years because of the commitment others made and the revival that happened on campus."

Tim talked, too, about his recent lengthy bout with a viral infection and the extensive tests he had to endure before he finally recovered.

"I felt like God had deserted me," he said. "I began to ask why God was putting me through these tests again. It started to defeat my faith and my whole outlook on God. But then I began to realize God wanted me to depend on Him to bring me through these times I struggle."

God *has* brought each one of us through these times when we struggle, but we are not the only family who has walked through the fire. After the first edition of this book was published, I received letters and phone calls from parents facing the complexities of raising a child with epilepsy or one who was hyperactive or who experienced both disabilities like our son.

Doctors told us hyperactive children outgrow their impulsive behavior. Even so, I had talked with many mothers whose children's hyperactivity turned into belligerent rebellion as they became teens and young adults. I didn't have many real answers for these mothers. There are still no simple solutions, and I can only share how we have been helped the most throughout these past nineteen years.

First, God led us to seek professional help. When we have children, we think raising them will be as instinctive as walking or eating. But when our children have special needs, we need specialized counseling. Counseling helped us gain perspective. It gave us tools to enable us to parent our son. It showed us where we needed to change, but it also reaffirmed us when we were doing our best.

God also led us to specific answers. We discovered Tim needed to avoid certain foods, petrochemicals, paint, and smog. These allergens lowered his threshold to seizures and increased his hyperactivity. They were not *the cure,* but they have made a significant difference over the past six years since we closed the final chapter of this book.

God taught us to support Tim's strengths and compensate for his disabilities. We have encouraged him in his mechanical skill, even when I cringe to see his work clothes and shoes saturated with black grease. He has overhauled motorcycle and Volkswagen engines and is now restoring his "Bug." When Tim struggled with school and wanted to quit, we reminded him that excellence in academics is not the mark of success or failure in life, but finishing the race is.

Finally, God moved us to pray and impressed numerous friends and people we have never met to pray with us. During our whirlwind season, when troubles rose in thick dust clouds and darkened our vision, we felt like Job who cried out for the Almighty to answer him. Our way had been hidden; we were hedged in. Why did God remain silent so long?

Now I look back and see how God answered us in His time and guided us in the way He knew best for us. Our family has seen God's caring presence in our lives in ways we never would have if we hadn't been through these experiences.

As with Job, God has answered our family out of the whirlwind. With Job we can say:

> I know that You can do all things and that no thought *or* purpose of Yours can be restrained *or* thwarted. I had heard of You [only] by the hearing of the ear; but now my [spiritual eye] sees You (Job 42:2,5, *AMP*).